GW01418670

The Story of the

Penny Farthing Reminiscence Centre

An exciting guide to help you set up your own memory room

by

Fiona Mahoney

DipCOT, SROT, MBAOT, ITEC, BFP

Published by:

The Somerset Virtual College NHS Publications

Dunkirk Memorial House

Minehead Road, Bishops Lydeard

Taunton, Somerset

TA4 3BT

Tel: 01823 431259

Copyright © Fiona Mahoney 2003

All rights reserved
No part of this publication may
be reproduced, stored in a retrieval
system, or transmitted in any form or
by any means electronic, mechanical,
photocopying, recording or otherwise,
without the prior permission
of the copyright holder.

A CIP catalogue record for this book
is available from the British Library

ISBN 0 9544475 1 4

Designed and Printed by
Colourtone Print and Graphics

Somerset Virtual College NHS Publications

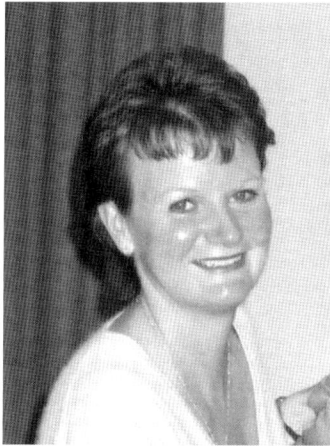

Fiona Mahoney, born in 1959, qualified as an occupational therapist in 1980 from St Loyes School of occupational therapy, Exeter. She has worked in both physical and mental health; her first job working with the elderly at Summerlands Hospital, Yeovil, Somerset. Fiona gained a promotion to become the rheumatology occupational therapist at Musgrove Park Hospital, Taunton, Somerset. Here she instigated and set up the joint protection group and the Taunton branch of Arthritis Care. Fiona through this branch of her work realised the need for a shop / demon- stration centre and left the NHS in 1986 to set up her own medical equipment company "Domestic and Medical Aids / The Making Life Easier Centre". In 1994 the company was divided up and sold and Fiona and her husband Ken chose to continue working only in the field of stairlifts and this continues to date as DMA Stairlifts.

Having an interest in complementary therapy and having had experienced successful results herself following Bells Palsy, Fiona decided in 1994 to train as a reflexologist. She left DMA Stairlifts in the capable hands of her husband and took up a post as reflexologist at Warwick House Medical Centre. Throughout the next few years she qualified as a Bach Flower Practitioner and worked also at the Somerset Nuffield Hospital in both complementary therapies and as their bank occupational therapist.

In 1995 Fiona went back working for the NHS at Stratfield House, Wellington, Somerset, this time within the field of mental health for the Somerset Partnership NHS and Social Care Trust. Her job was working with the elderly mentally ill and it was during the next few years that her interest grew and developed within the field of remini- scence. By 1999 she had fulfilled her dream to set up a place to preserve and stimulate memories in Wellington called the Penny Farthing Remini- scence Centre. This is the story of how that dream became reality.

CONTENTS

THE STORY OF THE PENNY FARTHING REMINISCENCE ROOM

DEDICATION

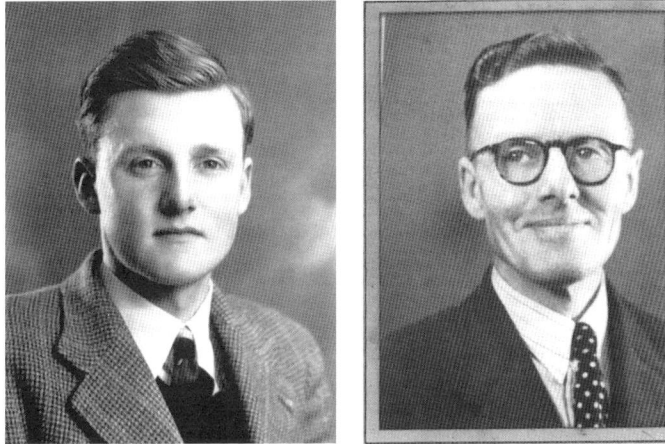

This book is dedicated to my adorable Dad
whom I loved and miss so much. I know he
would have been so proud of me.
Also to my precious grandfather 'Gaffer' who
became like a father to me when he prematurely
lost his only son (my father).

The reminiscence room is said by many to have a
calming and peaceful influence and I believe both my
Dad and Gaffer have been with me and will continue
to be with me throughout my work in reminiscence.

Introduction – A Reminiscence Adventure

To begin with an embryo of an idea and turn it into reality gives one such a feeling of complete satisfaction and immense pride.

This is the story of how the Penny Farthing Reminiscence Centre was formed, shaped and developed to provide Wellington in Somerset with an excellent community resource for reminiscence. Writing it all has also proved to be a most worthy and satisfying reminiscence exercise for me.

It all started many years ago when I had taken a change in my career and decided to sell my equipment company The Making Life Easier Centre and return to occupational therapy within an NHS Trust in the field of mental health for older people.

Although reminiscence had been a subject briefly touched on during my training, little did I know it would become my "buzz" word for the next few years and the foreseeable future.

My interest soon began to develop and because of this I began to expand my knowledge, reading books and generally becoming more aware of how beneficial and therapeutic reminiscence can be, not only for the older person, but also for anyone of any age or walk of life.

I heard about Age Exchange, the national reminiscence centre in Blackheath, London and planned a visit.

From the moment I stepped into Age Exchange in London,

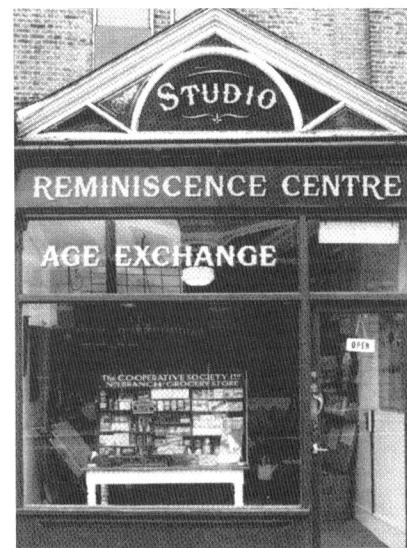

and consequently stepped back in time, I realised that reminiscence and I had something to share.

My interest in reminiscence deepened and widened and my enthusiasm on my return to work encouraged me to start using it more widely in the therapeutic field with the elderly mentally ill.

I started to run regular sessions. Each time my eyes became wider by the reaction and satisfaction some of the patients were obviously gaining from these groups.

To run a group successfully you need a co-facilitator to ensure there is always someone available to focus on one individual should the need arise and for each session another member of staff would start to enjoy the reminiscence work and so throughout the months / years the 'buzz' was beginning to spread.

One of the ideas borrowed from Age Exchange was the gathering and collating of memorabilia and placing these in memory boxes.

We all started to have a fascination with junk shops, people's garages and old lofts.

Reminiscence started more and more to become part of everyday life. Soon we had all collected memorabilia for six boxes and so we recorded all the items and included in each box a file explaining how to use the box with ideas for therapeutic activities and some background information on reminiscence.

Soon we were over-flowing with knick-knacks and artefacts of all shapes and sizes and it was obvious a more permanent and functional resource was required to allow reminiscence to grow and develop.

Excited by the thousands of "trinkets" - the idea to set up a reminiscence centre was born.

This book has been put together to excite and encourage you to do the same and to help you to realise that it is not as complex or financially crippling as you may imagine. However it is initially very labour intensive, needs a sense of commitment, motivation and drive and from this you will receive a real sense of achievement and the 'buzz' that reminiscence is able to give.

I have divided the book up into chapters to provide you with lots of basic facts and ideas, tips on things to do and not to do and a blueprint to guide you through the reminiscence adventure.

Remember nothing is set in stone, these are only my ideas and can be easily adapted and changed. Hopefully it will enthuse you and allow you to step on to the first rung to help you set up your own reminiscence room.

I wish you every success and don't forget: It's the 'buzz' that keeps you driving on.

Trinkets

TRINKETS = Key to success

T = Trust your own judgement

R = Run with your ideas

I = Involve others

N = Never weaken

K = Keep smiling

E = Enthuse at all times

T = Test out new ideas

S = Succeed against all odds

1.Were these things given to me for a reason?

My Grandfather, fondly known to all as Gaffer, was in his 96th year and finding living at home alone a daily struggle. He decided to leave his 2-bedroom bungalow in Widmer End, Buckinghamshire, where he had lived ever since my Gran had died in 1978 and move into a nursing home where his loneliness and dependence would heighten.

He had declined moving in with our family as he felt he would become too much of a burden. I am sure he regretted this decision, as I did when his life started to ebb away in the claustrophobic surroundings of an institution.

Once he had chosen a few precious possessions, a life times worth of memorabilia was packed into a few cardboard boxes and transported with him to fill a room that already had a bed, wardrobe, chair and basin. A ragged cheap seaside print clinging to a frame precariously hung over the bed.

This heart-breaking experience I am convinced shortened his life and prevented him from reaching the grand old age of 100 that we had all felt would be of no great trial for a man with such dignity, pride and determination.

His chosen possessions carefully arranged in his small room approximately 12' x 10', he asked my sister and I to clear his bungalow and choose any items we wanted and the rest was to be auctioned.

The weekend was full of mixed feelings, the highs and lows one experiences through reminiscence, a sense that an era had ended. All those exciting memories of childhood when my dad had been alive and the realisation that the Gaffer who had often been strict and occasionally scary was actually a romantic sentimental old thing who had boxes of old love letters tied with ribbons, wedding cake frippery and dog-eared photographs tucked in wallets and diaries.

He obviously adored my Gran and beautiful photographs and touching prayers were found throughout his possessions.

He suddenly became a different kind of gentleman, whom although he was still alive was having his life analysed and torn apart and his secrets made public without his knowledge. I wanted him to be excited coming across these memorabilia. I wanted him to be saying "Oh do you remember this" or "What about that?". I suppose if I am honest I really wanted him to be resting in peace. I felt guilty visiting him in a place so alien to him, the independent Gaffer I so loved and adored.

We spent hours slowly and meticulously picking our way through the drawers, cupboards, suitcases and old rusty tins in the garage.

We had organised a skip to be available and we had a van to take any furniture or larger items we wanted to preserve as a family heirloom and treasure.

We had a limited time of two days to clear a lifetime of treasures and we were consequently forced to speed up the process and hurriedly jam things into boxes, promising to read or investigate them in greater detail as soon as we got home.

Too many memories, too many items to spend the appropriate time they deserved on each valuable piece. Looking back on it now it all seems rather amusing. My sister, Trina would ask whether she could have a piece of silver or this lovely desk or beautiful hand painted vase and I was more excited and thrilled by the rusty old oxo tin or the box of antiquated tools stashed in a cobweb swamped corner of the garage.

The old passports dating back to 1923 with a most glamorous Elizabeth Symon (his wife, my gran) pictured in a typical 1920's hat with stamps from numerous countries such as Switzerland.

DESCRIPTION OF BEARER.	DESCRIPTION OF WIFE OF BEARER.
Age 18. Profession Student	Age _____ Profession _____
Place & date of birth Chiswick 9 April 1902	Place & date of birth _____
Maiden name if widow or married woman travelling singly } _____	Maiden name _____
Height 5 feet 1 inches	Height _____ feet _____ inches
Forehead Straight Eyes Brown	Forehead _____ Eyes _____
Nose Short Mouth Small	Nose _____ Mouth _____
Chin Prominent Colour of Hair dark brown	Chin _____ Colour of Hair _____
Complexion Fresh Face Round	Complexion _____ Face _____
Any special peculiarities Large mole on left cheek	Any special peculiarities _____
National Status British born subject	

PARTICULARS OF CHILDREN UNDER THE AGE OF 16 YEARS.

Name	Age	Sex

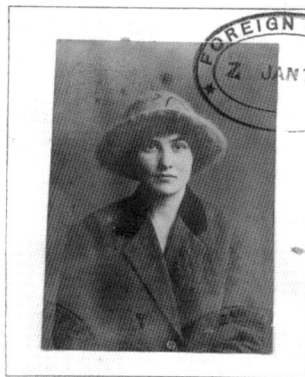

PHOTOGRAPH OF BEARER.   PHOTOGRAPH OF WIFE.

FOREIGN OFFICE
Z JAN 1921

SIGNATURE OF BEARER.   SIGNATURE OF WIFE.

* E. S. Symon.

13

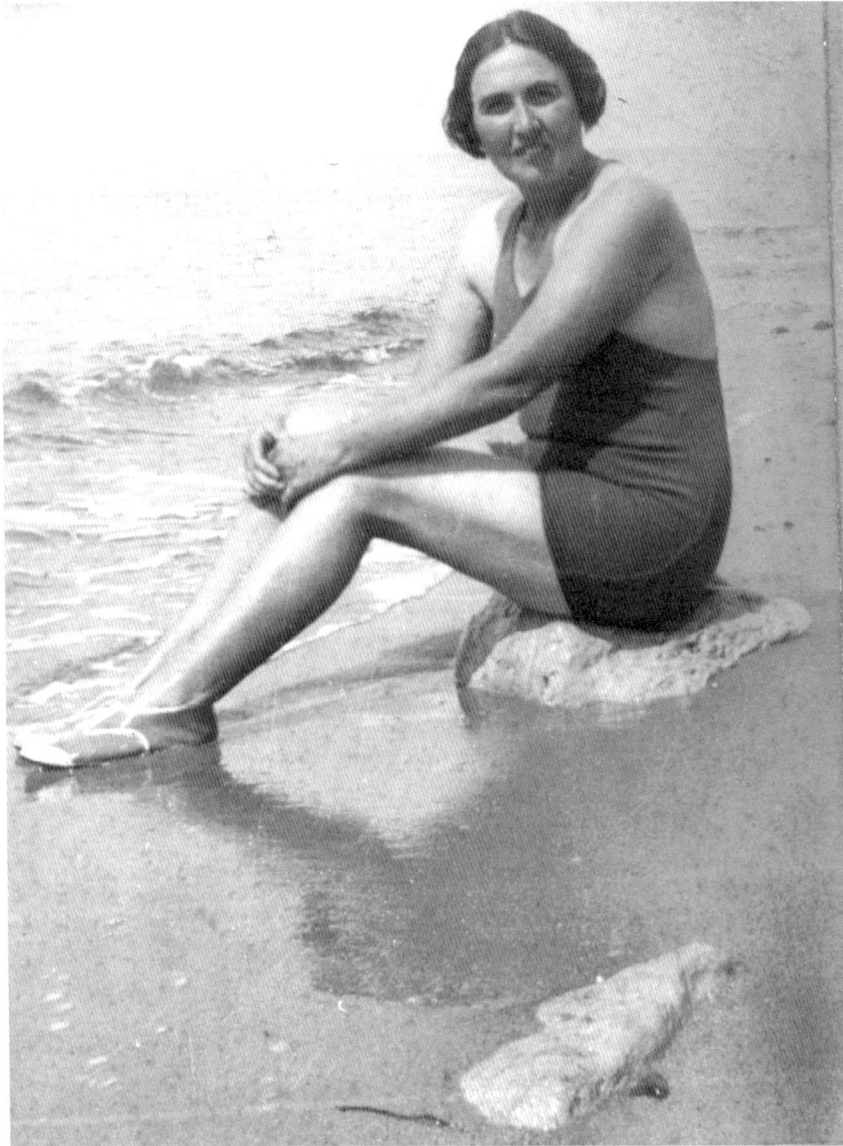

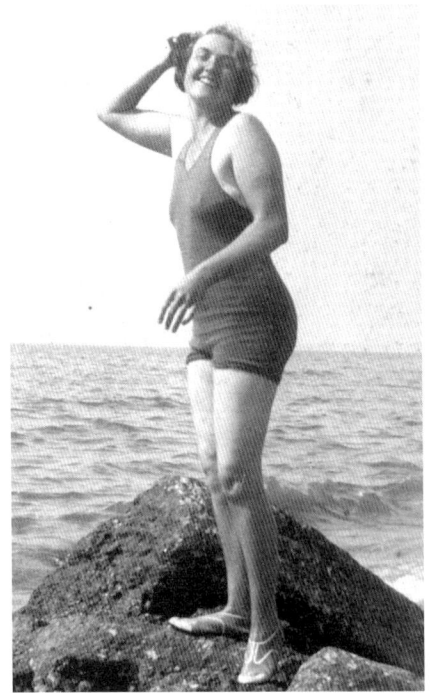

Some wonderful pictures of my gran in her swimwear posing seductively against a rock, something I had definitely never seen before.

A medal, letter and certificate thanking Gaffer for being in the Civil Defence, transfer and air raid documentation. Plus envelopes with broken pieces of submarine etc.

WE DESIRE on behalf of His Majesty's Government to thank you in common with all others who came forward so readily during the crisis and gave their services to the Country in the capacity of Special Constables.

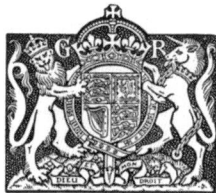

Stanley Baldwin
PRIME MINISTER.

W Joynson Hicks
HOME SECRETARY.

Downing Street,
May, 1926.

To _____

METROPOLITAN SPECIAL CONSTABULARY RESERVE.

AS.16950

CERTIFICATE of* { Discharge / Transfer to Reserve / Disembodiment / Demobilization } on Demobilization.   Army Form Z. 21.

N.B.—Any person finding this Certificate is requested to forward it in an unstamped envelope to the Secretary, War Office, London, S.W. 1.

WARNING.—If this Certificate is lost a duplicate cannot be issued. You should therefore on no account part with it or forward it by post when applying for a situation.

Regtl. No. G/37307. Rank Pte.

Names in full Wilkinson Arthur Joseph
(Surname first)

Unit and Regiment or Corps from which *Discharged / Transferred to Reserve   Depot Royal Sussex Rgt

Attested on the 4. 7. 191 7

Called up for Service on the 6. 3. 191 8

For Honorable Artillery Coy
(Here state Regiment or Corps to which first appointed)

Also served in ...... Nil

Only Regiments or Corps in which the Soldier served since August 4th, 1914, are to be stated. If inapplicable, this space is to be ruled through in ink and initialled.

†Medals and Decorations awarded during present engagement   Nil
Authorised prior to 11th Novr. 1918

*Has / Has not } served Overseas on Active Service.

Place of Rejoining in case of emergency }   SHORNCLIFFE   Medical Category A1

Specialist Military qualifications }   Year of birth 1900

He is* { Discharged / Transferred to Army Reserve / Disembodied / Demobilized } on 9. 2. 191 20

In consequence of Demobilization.

for .... Signature and Rank.

Officer i/c No. 2 Infantry Records. HOUNSLOW (Place).

* Strike out whichever is inapplicable.   + The word "Nil" to be inserted when necessary.

(23744). Wt. W 1439—P.P. 2449. 600m. 6/19. D & S. (E 1256.)

In the years when our Country was in mortal danger

ARTHUR JOSEPH WILKINSON

who served 6 July 1942 – 31 December 1944 gave generously of his time and powers to make himself ready for her defence by force of arms and with his life if need be.

George R.I.

THE HOME GUARD

16

RICKMANSWORTH URBAN DISTRICT COUNCIL.

AIR RAID PRECAUTIONS.

This is to certify that A. J. WILKINSON has been appointed one of the Local Authority's Air Raid Wardens and is authorised to carry out the duties of that office on behalf of the Local Authority.

C. G. RANSOME WILLIAMS,
Clerk of the Council.

A.R.27A. SHAW & SONS LTD., FETTER LANE, E.C.4. E 80984

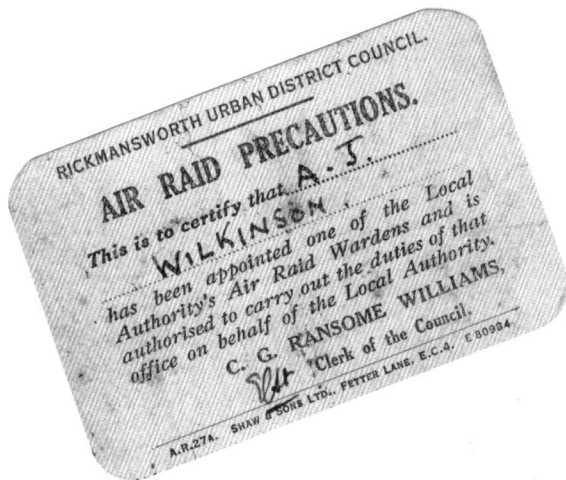

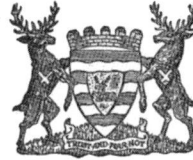

COUNTY OF HERTFORD

LIEUTENANCY OFFICE,

HERTFORD.

Date March 1946

DEAR Mr Wilkinson

It is a great privilege to me now that the Civil Defence Organization has been disbanded to convey to you this expression of appreciation for the service you have so ably rendered towards the general defence of this Country.

It must be a satisfaction to you and a legitimate cause for pride to know that the local authority and the general public will long remember with gratitude the unfailing trust and confidence they vested in you during the long period of the war.

His Majesty's Lieutenant
of the County of Hertford.

17

The lecture notes my gran had written about childhood foods.

Did you, I wonder, suffer the same awful agonies in childhood as we did over our food at the family meal times? Looking back to those sessions at the nursery table, when sloppy burnt milk puddings arrived in enamel pie-dishes, and there were ~~interms~~ seemingly unending fights with Nanny or Mother to choke down suffocating spoonsful of the rapidly cooling mess, each mouthful hastier than the last. Were you told as we were, that there were many poor little boys and girls who would only be too glad to have such a good meal? My childish mind could never grapple with the answer that came back when you suggested giving it to the said boys and girls, and asked " Why should I eat it if they needed food", " Just because—" was all the Grown-Ups would say, "now hurry up", and the struggle would go on.

Tripe was another colourless dish which seemed to make a frequent entrance, and it was as flavourless as pale. The Grown-Ups had an idea that childish stomachs could absorb quantities of these revolting things and had no idea in the early nineteen hundreds of giving anything special or tempting to a youngster. At breakfast the too porridge always seemed to be full of knots that stuck in one's throat, and to be told that luke warm grey mass was "good for you" did not seem a

great start for a child's day. Of
course we've gone a long way in
domestic comfort since then and
my family has never known the
smell of a smoky, dull and sulky
dining room fire ~~for their~~ at breakfast time,
nor indeed have they had to practise
the arts of evading the bathroom
and ~~hand~~ face flannel, ~~not~~ because
~~there was only cold water in the tap,~~
~~or a can of tepid water~~ because
you had delayed too long pretending
you were an explorer, or a fine lady
going out to call, instead of wrestling
with buttons on your liberty bodice
and flannel petticoats. Central
heating, good gas fires and a
wider knowledge of simple cooking can

and sensing have made life for the
modern child much more idyllic, and
lucky is the small person who has
pretty dishes and an imaginative
mamma to provide exciting ~~food~~,
and who has the wisdom to place only
as much as the child will eat in
front of him . Of course there were
favourite meals
~~a few days when~~ one enjoyed
400
~~meals~~ very much, even in the bad
old days. To come in from a sharp
winter's walk and find lovely
lentil soup for mid-day dinner,
and if Nanny was in a good
mood you were allowed to stick
fingers of bread across the plate to
look like the white posts in the old
house pond which you had seen

that morning; when there was steamed suet pudding covered in hot ~~golden~~ syrup, or perhaps a chicken[26]. But these days were golden occasions, and ~~looking backs~~ in spite of ration cuts and shortages, I am more than happy to be where I am, and do not sigh for "the good old days"

509

Elizabeth Wilkinson, Guest writer, remembers the food troubles of her childhood, and decides in spite of rations, that present day menus are better.

¶

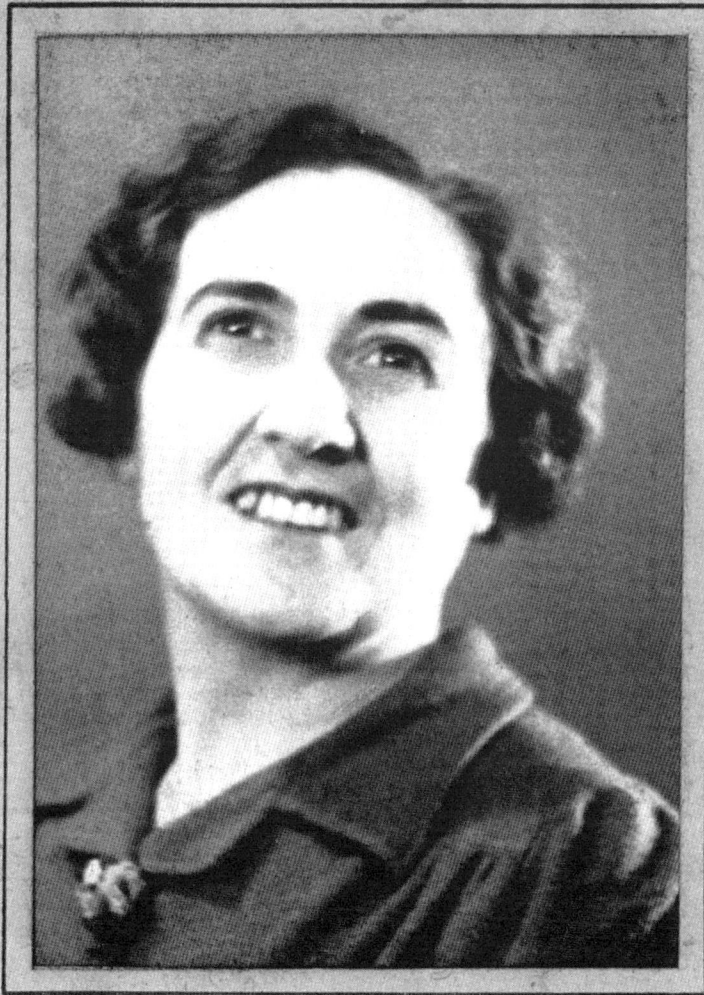

Probably my most valuable find was a rusty old biscuit tin that narrowly missed its demise in the skip. Feeling heavy I hurriedly prised it open to discover nearly 100 glass negatives all carefully preserved in their thick cardboard boxes with separate tissue paper envelopes and all marked individually with date and subject.

Initially they were an exciting find but questionable as to their usage, although subsequently their worth and usage has been tremendous.

A photographer, Jesper Nors who soon after this find was carrying out a residency at Stratfield House in Wellington was looking for projects to cover for his commission piece.

I hesitantly showed the negatives to him and asked if he thought the faded images would reproduce. He wasn't sure but agreed to take them

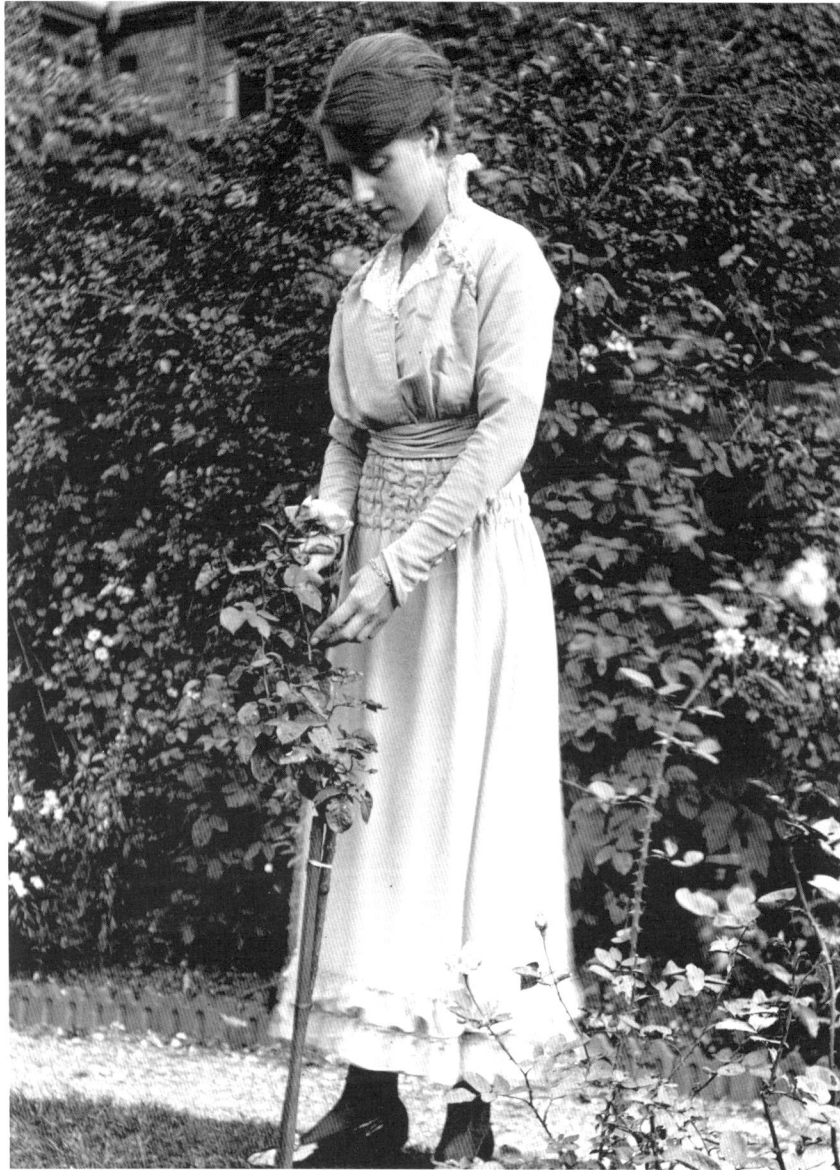

away and see what he could do with them.

To mine and his amazement the reproduction and clarity of these glass plates was fantastic. Every last detail in black and white was clear for all to see and he decided to enlarge some to use as a commission piece for the hospital. These now have pride of place in the Penny Farthing Reminiscence Centre.

It all became quite a revelation to see my grandfather as a boy and great grandparents and his sisters Olive and Dorothy, the latter whom I have very fond memories as a beautifully preserved old lady. Her photograph when she was about 17 years old, so elegant and charming.

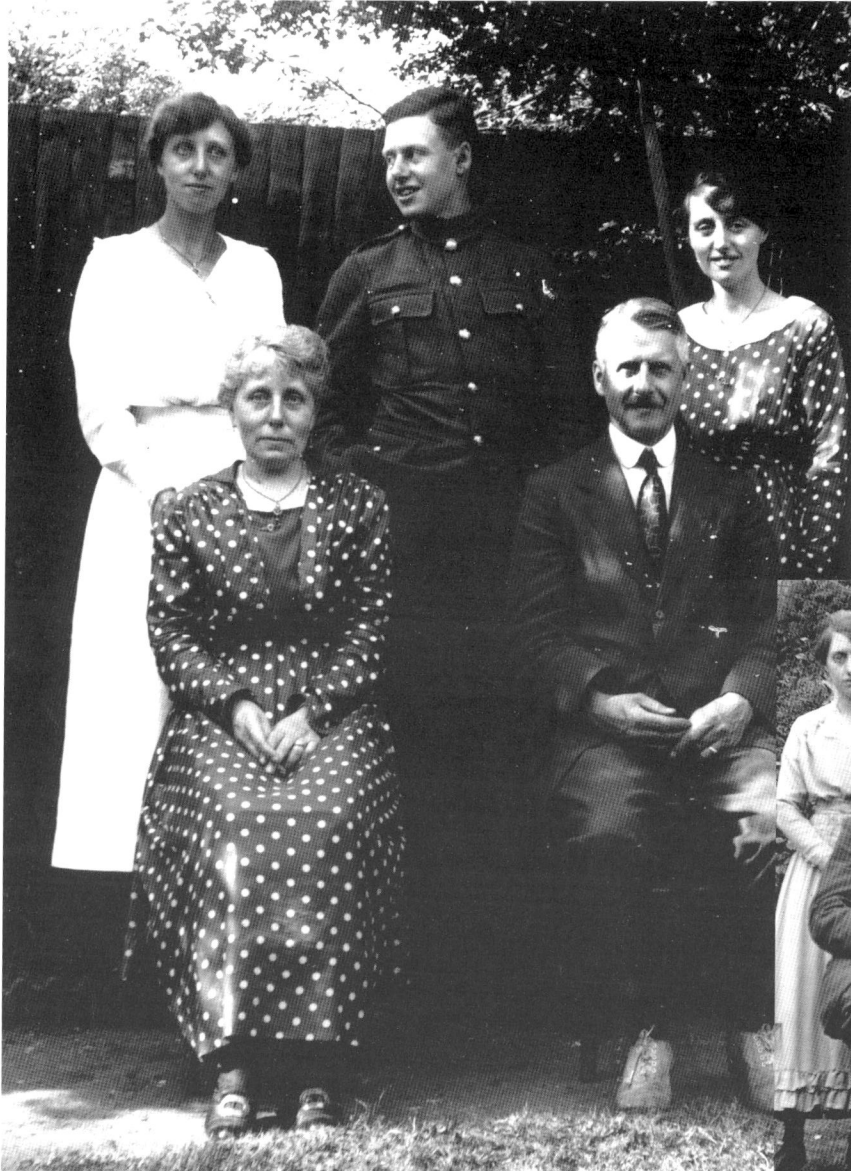
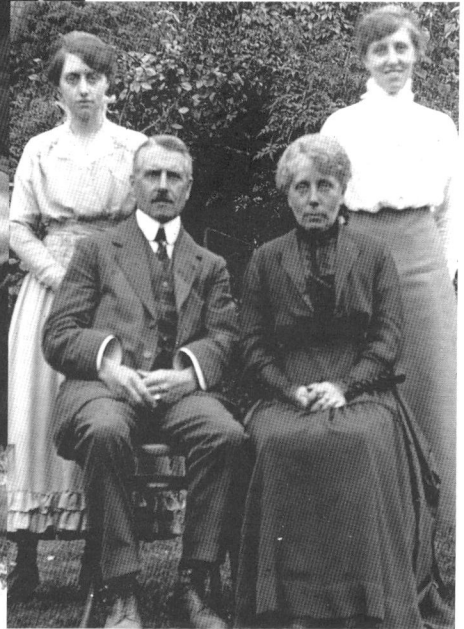

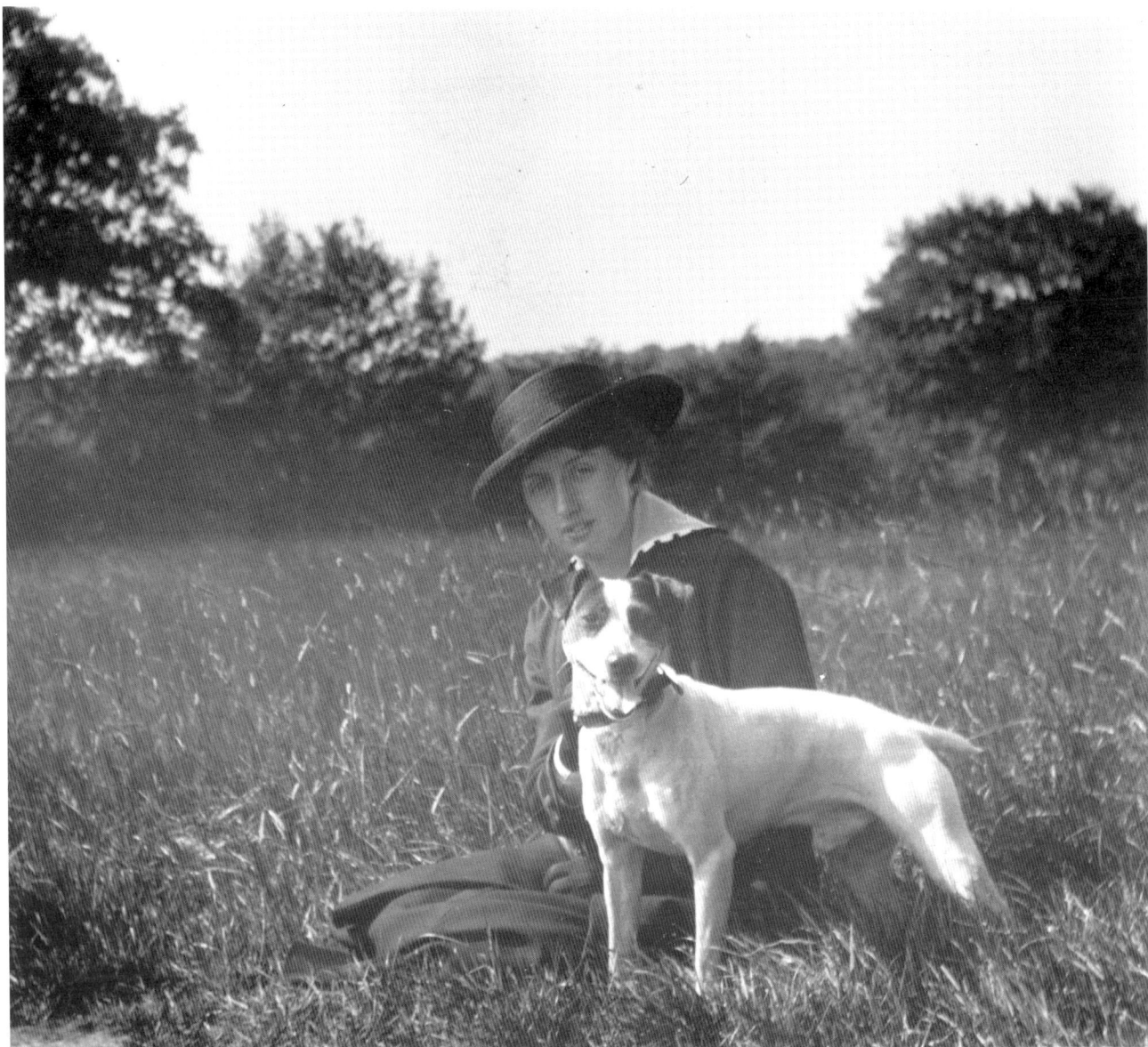

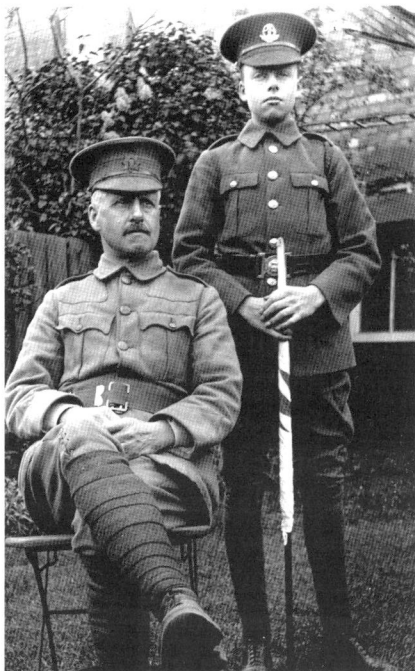

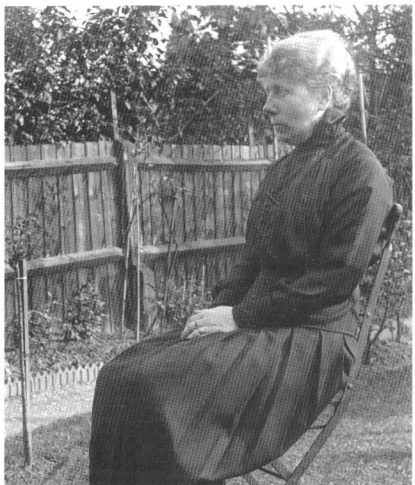

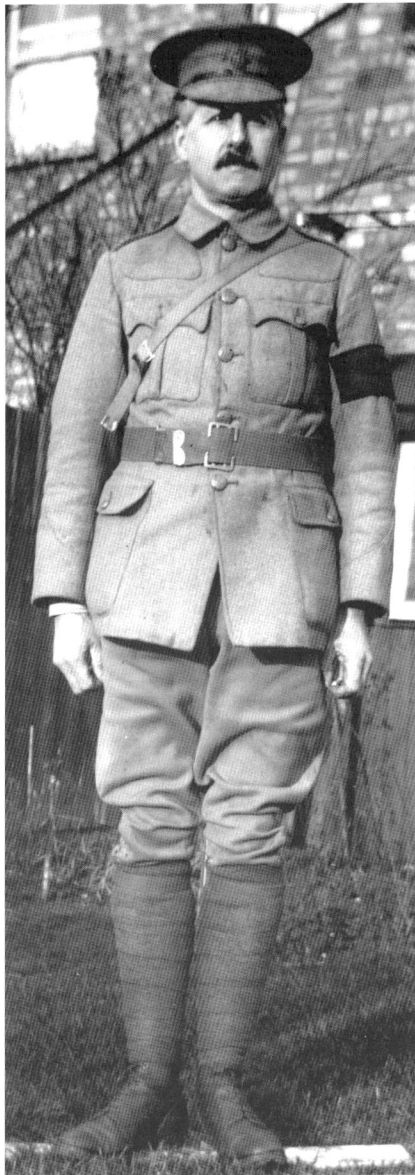

From stirrup pump and tin helmets to candle snuffers and cribbage boards every piece of memorabilia is now not just stored in an old cardboard box and left in a forgotten attic but it makes up the whole infrastructure of the Penny Farthing Reminiscence Centre. It is there to be looked at, touched and used as hands on multi sensory experience, for people of all ages and all walks of life.

The memories of Granny and Gaffer continue to live on in the room and their photographs look down on all those who choose to share these treasures with them.

2. Quest for a suitable venue

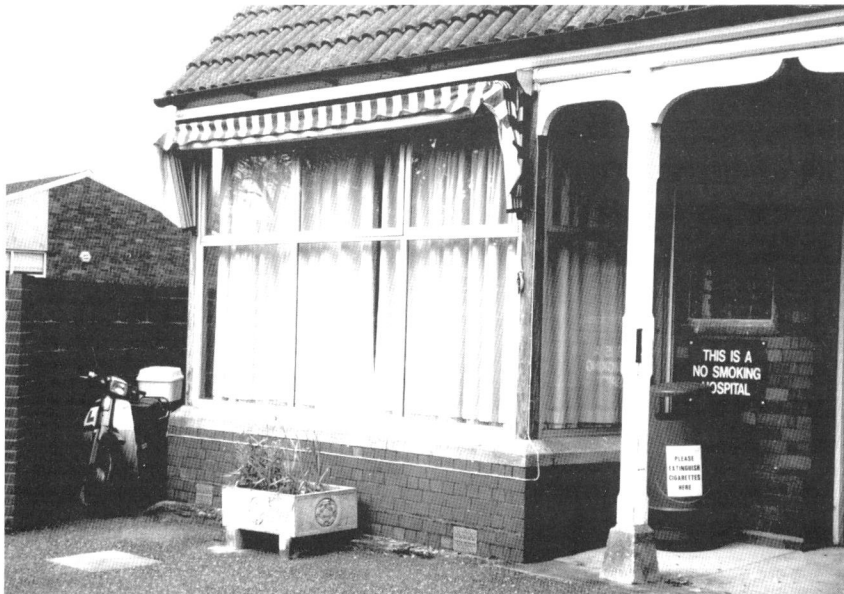

Large or small, in town or in the hospital? These were the first questions buzzing around in my head. I originally had visions of a coffee shop type place, situated centrally in Wellington Town which would be very visible with an attractive frontage, passed by regular shoppers who would stop by for a coffee and delve into a memory box. I had imagined it being under the town clock entwined in the labyrinth of shops in the Cornhill Parade. But I think this was a fantasy world I had fleetingly drifted into.

The centre had to be easily manageable, probably by myself as I would be unlikely to find a manager or volunteers to oversee and be responsible for its management and be as passionate about the place as me. After all it was my baby and so it would need caring for and nurturing.

One day I was sitting in the office scribbling some notes when I quietly looked around the room and inspired by what I saw decided that it would be a most suitable room and ideal to be converted into a front

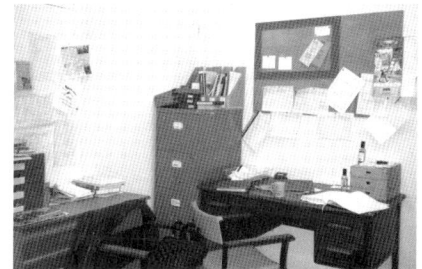

room in 30's and 40's style.

My imagination started to run wild. I could visualise every last nook and cranny and soon the hand that was supposed to be writing up medical notes was hastily scribbling on a scrap of crumpled paper. Swirling around in my chair, my head darting this way and that and jumping up and down from my chair to view the room from an alternative angle, I had soon sketchily planned the new Penny Farthing Reminiscence Centre.

Brilliant! It was integral within the hospital. It could be easily staffed and used by patients and staff alike for both the physical and mental health trusts that shared the grounds of Wellington Cottage Hospital and Stratfield House.

Solved! No need to walk the streets of Wellington any longer, I had found the ideal spot and it had been right under my nose all the time.

My elation soon turned to confusion and the problems started to flood my mind.

Firstly this was the main office and we had no alternative place to go and secondly I would have to convince everyone that this mind-blowing idea had some purpose, value and useful reason to even be considered, let alone become reality.

So my next quest was to look for an alternative place to house the office.

Regular reminiscence sessions were being held in the day hospital and we had started to collect additional small items of memorabilia.

An old pine Welsh dresser had been re-positioned into one corner with a couple of armchairs and a coffee table and a few reminiscence books and old ornaments were perfectly positioned on the shelves to show their great beauty.

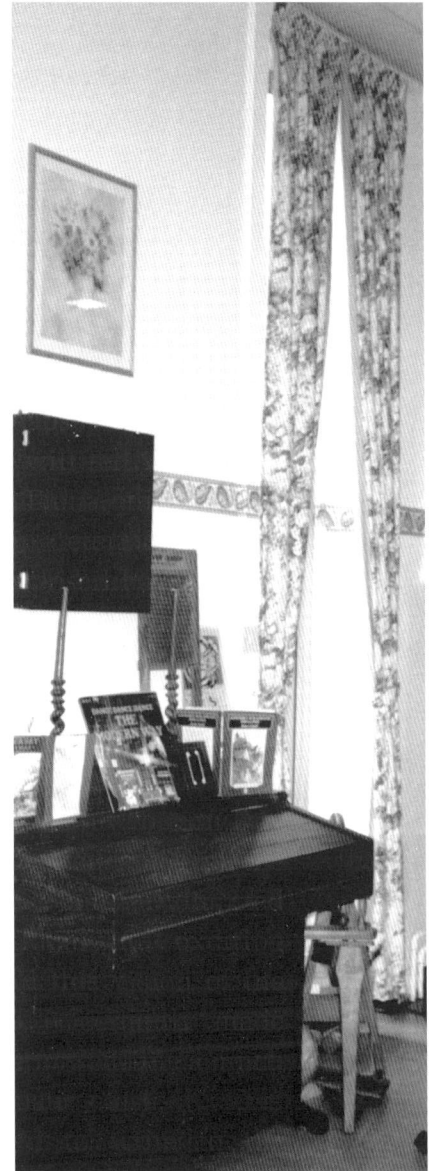

An old organ formed one dividing wall of the reminiscence area and the folded up table tennis table formed the second dividing wall. Posters, postcards and a couple of "oldish" looking pictures were re-located to join the reminiscence area and two barley twist candlesticks proudly stood on the organ either side of some old sheet music.

Yes, it looked quite good and yes, it was at last making a small statement about reminiscence and yes, it prompted me to start purchasing boxes from Home Base to collect themed items such as dressing up and looking good, going to work and shopping.

By gathering items in boxes it started to provide a focus as to the type of items we really required and helped to make it easier for individual staff to use.

Although this designated area had some advantages it also had some disadvantages. It was for example, never as private or secluded as I had imagined. The noise from the adjoining day hospital was a constant hum in the background and often other people would wander aimlessly in whilst you were half way through a thrilling story of someone's past. It all started to become a little frustrating so the campaign begun to really get the show on the road and fulfil my dream. Let's create the reminiscence centre in its own private and secluded environment.

I initially spoke with my unit manager Tracey Bright who had originally been in on the genesis of this idea and of having somewhere in the South West. We had excitedly discussed it, giggled about it and surpassed everyone's fantasy over a cup of coffee at Hammersmith Bus Station, having just been fired with enthusiasm at a visit to Age Exchange London. So I knew that I would have a favourable response from this corner of the ring. But when the other corner, namely the Trust, said sorry we have no money to convert any offices let alone rebuild a new one, I felt momentarily jilted, but as any of my close friends or colleagues will tell you if you say "no" to Fiona, it just makes her more determined. It's funny I suppose I have always been like this through life the eternal optimist, being a true Taurean, bull in a china shop and stubborn to the end. So at a complete crossroads I had to decide which way to turn. My hours of writing notes in the office were beautifully tainted with irrational but exciting ideas. I had this vision of the future and it certainly made note and report writing a much more fascinating task.

I decided to write to the League of Friends to see if I

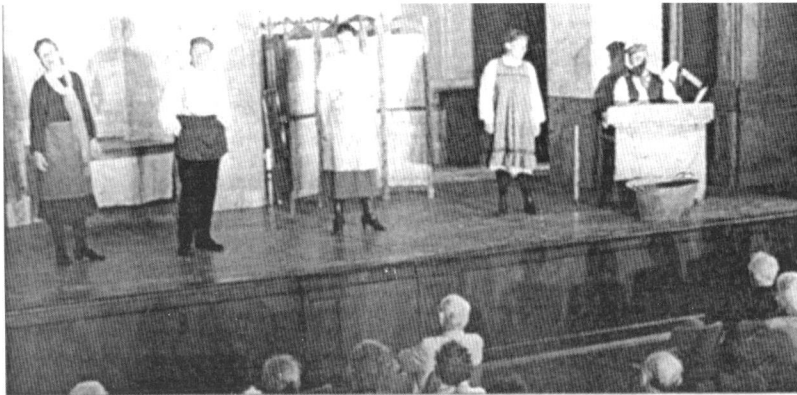

MEMORIES were stirred of how life used to be before the National Health Service when Age Exchange Theatre presented a musical *Can we Afford the Doctor?* to a large audience in Great Hall, Wellington.

The 75-minute play explores visits to and from the doctor, health care in hospitals and clinics as well as some of the gruelling home cures. A mixture of medical memories, music and mirth was dispensed

Life before the NHS

alongside the more serious story of the emerging health care system in the 1940s and 50s.

Among the audience were residents of local nursing homes and members of local organisations who were delighted to talk about their own reminiscences to members of the cast at the end of the production.

The play is currently on a national tour to coincide with the celebrations for the 50th anniversary of the NHS.

The visit was arranged by the Avalon Trust who run Stratfield House, for the elderly, mentally ill in Wellington.

Senior occupational therapist at Stratfield House, Fiona Mahoney said the trust were hoping to provide a special reminiscence room for residents and visitors and a bid was being made for a rural development grant. This play was very helpful towards this work and she was very grateful to Wellington School for the use of Great Hall.

could enthuse them. Within a fortnight I had a most encouraging reply inviting me to go and enlighten them at their next committee meeting in July. However there was a slightly disheartening footnote asking if I had asked the Trust for their financial assistance. Knowing that I had had a negative response, I prevented my emotions from roller-coasting to the floor and with my eternal optimist's hat on thought to my self, "Oh I'll get over that one some how". After all I had a month to think about it.

Prior to this important meeting I had arranged for a theatre group from Age Exchange in London to visit and present a reminiscence musical called 'Can we Afford the Doctor'. It was celebrating the 50 years of the NHS and was very aptly timed.

I sent invitations to all the local nursing and residential homes and advertised in the local Wellington Weekly. I had decided that the response to this event would seal my commitment or otherwise, as to the future and success for my new idea.

Using my contacts with my son's school, I arranged for the musical to be held in the Great Hall and Yes it was three quaters full. Everyone thoroughly enjoyed the show and my renewed confidence and excitement drove me on to plan my talk to the League of Friends.

I knew that once I started to talk about the project I would readily show my great passion for it but I had to ensure that I explained to those who were not so aware exactly what reminiscence could offer, to make them believe in its concept and therapeutic value.

To ensure this successful outcome I decided to lay out all the themed boxes in the day hospital with examples of work that had been carried out by the patients. Prior to my talk I took the committee on a guided tour around the room explaining what each box consisted of and how I could improve and develop upon these ideas in conjunction with a resource room. I used the small cordoned off area as an example of what we were attempting to achieve with limited space and resources and then when I had their full attention during my talk, I compared the areas with the benefits of having a specialist and focused environment for reminiscence only.

Having been so enthusiastic that I could hardly sit still in my seat and having had to restrain myself from gabbling incoherently. I finally admitted that I had already approached the Trust and explained that their finances were not able to stretch to such an ambitious and unproven project.

I left and waited with bated breath for a reply. The letter from the league of friends arrived and this gave me hope but not confirmation. I realised there was some concern due to it being an office relocation and funds were not normally used for this purpose, however in this instance circumstances were very different in that it was the only available space in the hospital, even though at present it wasn't actually available and the project would be a non starter if I was unable to obtain funding. Well that's what they think!

A telephone call out of the blue and we are green for GO. The League of Friends said Yes and all that we needed now was to top up their funding with a little bit of fund raising and my dream would soon be realised. So a letter explaining my ideas and how it will be funded now had to be sent to the locality services manager and another green drove me forward to organise the Stratfield House Christmas Fayre.

The headline in the Wellington Weekly read "Bowled over by support for centre". I hadn't yet learnt that what ever you say, and even things you don't say, end up in speech marks. According to the papers I was bowled over by the tremendous support for the event, and yes I think at the time I could not believe the enthusiasm shown by members of the local community. However I also became known by the Wellington Weekly as the person who pioneered a scheme to " heal ", something I quickly had to rectify with the papers.

Success! We had raised £825.00 at the christmas fayre, a very pleasing result and the target was nearing success. Only £700 to go. But £700 is £700 when you haven't got it and so out came the keyboard and a few more letters were written to the local community, drug companies, schools, charities. The list was endless and a few companies came up trumps.

Nearing our final figure, it was time to check on the final plans we had drawn up for the new office and the builders moved in. A few changes to detail as we went along; a door to move, a window to lower.

Join us for hot punch &
a mince pie

@

STRATFIELD HOUSE CHRISTMAS FAYRE

Friday 4th December

6.00 - 8.00 pm

Carol Singing   Raffles   Father Christmas
Cakes/sweets   Lucky Dip
Chocoholics   White Elephant   Gifts
Plants   Table Decorations   Bottle Stall

All proceeds to New Reminiscence Centre

Then we were ready to move in.

With the sweet smell of new paint and the spongy new carpet the office was at last on the move, freeing up the space that was to become my living vision.

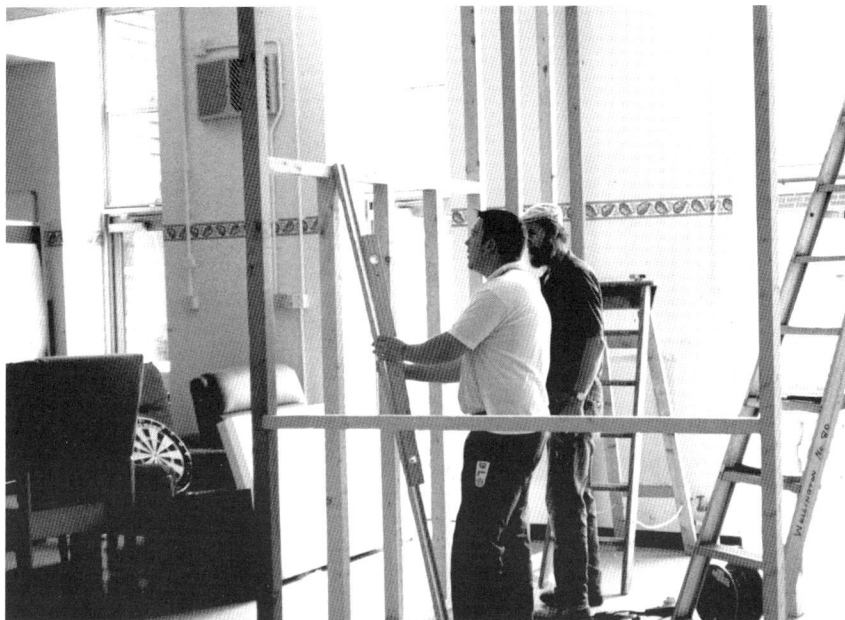

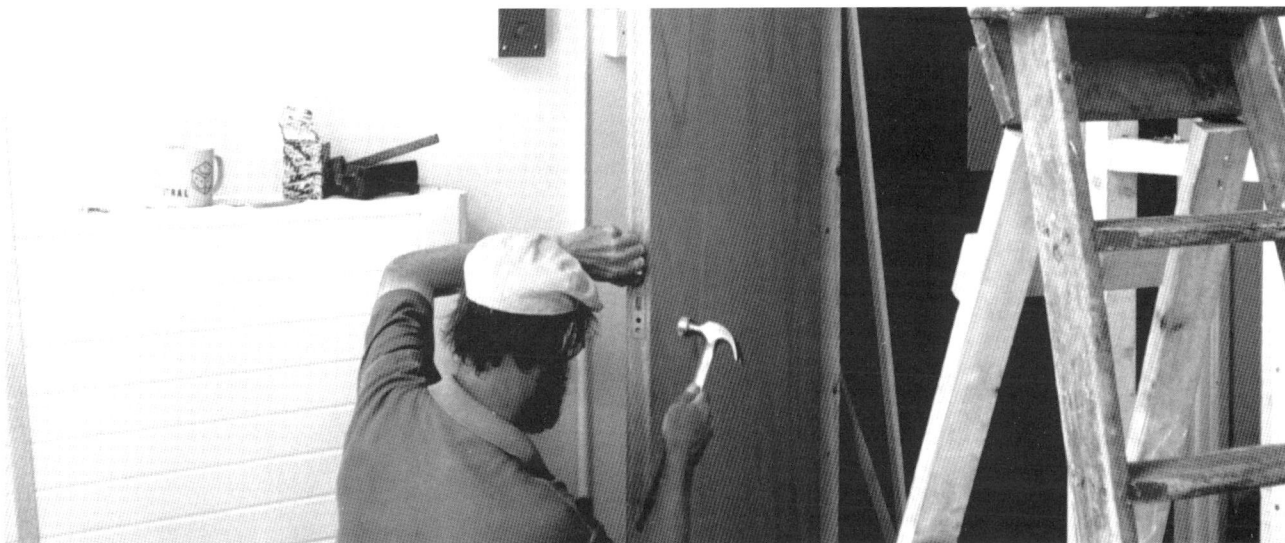

3. From office to centre

From books to bellows, mincers to mothballs, the new challenge had suddenly begun and I was faced with a totally blank canvas. Like every work of art the basic foundations and colours are very important prior to putting on the top finishing touches. The ideas had for a long time now been spinning helplessly out of control in my mind and it was now time to harness them and put paint to wall and bring my blank canvas to life.

A few months before we had been asked if we would like to be involved with Take Art and have an artist in residence at Stratfield House. Part of the remit would be to assist with the setting up of the new Reminiscence Centre.

"Fantastic", was my reply when asked to join the steering committee. From that moment on months of discussion groups, endless meetings and reams of CVS had to be ploughed through in order to find a suitable candidate who would be able to enhance the aesthetic pleasure of a hospital setting. A mighty task for any artist. The hardest problem was to actually find someone who was an artist and an artist in the eyes of the public. How do you choose when everyone's concept of art is so varied and extreme?

After a series of interviews a candidate was finally chosen who had expressed an interest in old memorabilia and was offered the residency.

Unfortunately her term with us was shorter than we had expected and I was finally bailed out by Lyn Ferguson a woman I had met at a dried flower party and who happened to be an interior designer and had been involved with some ideas for my own home.

Having brainstormed my ideas on to paper and sketched a very simplistic design on to card I showed them to the interior designer.

The main problem we faced was that the room had incredibly tall ceilings compared to the overall size and its height made it feel even smaller. Lyn brought in some swatches of heritage colours and made up a most stimulating colour board full of tissue paper, bows, ribbons, wallpaper samples, and magazine snippets. It was a work of art all of its own and as she explained we would not necessarily be using the exact materials or designs but the overall colour and effect would help us to progress forward with our ideas. She was right it really did work and soon the paint colours had been chosen, including changing all the woodwork from brown to racing green or should I say Light Brunswick Green, chosen from the Dulux range of Victorian colours.

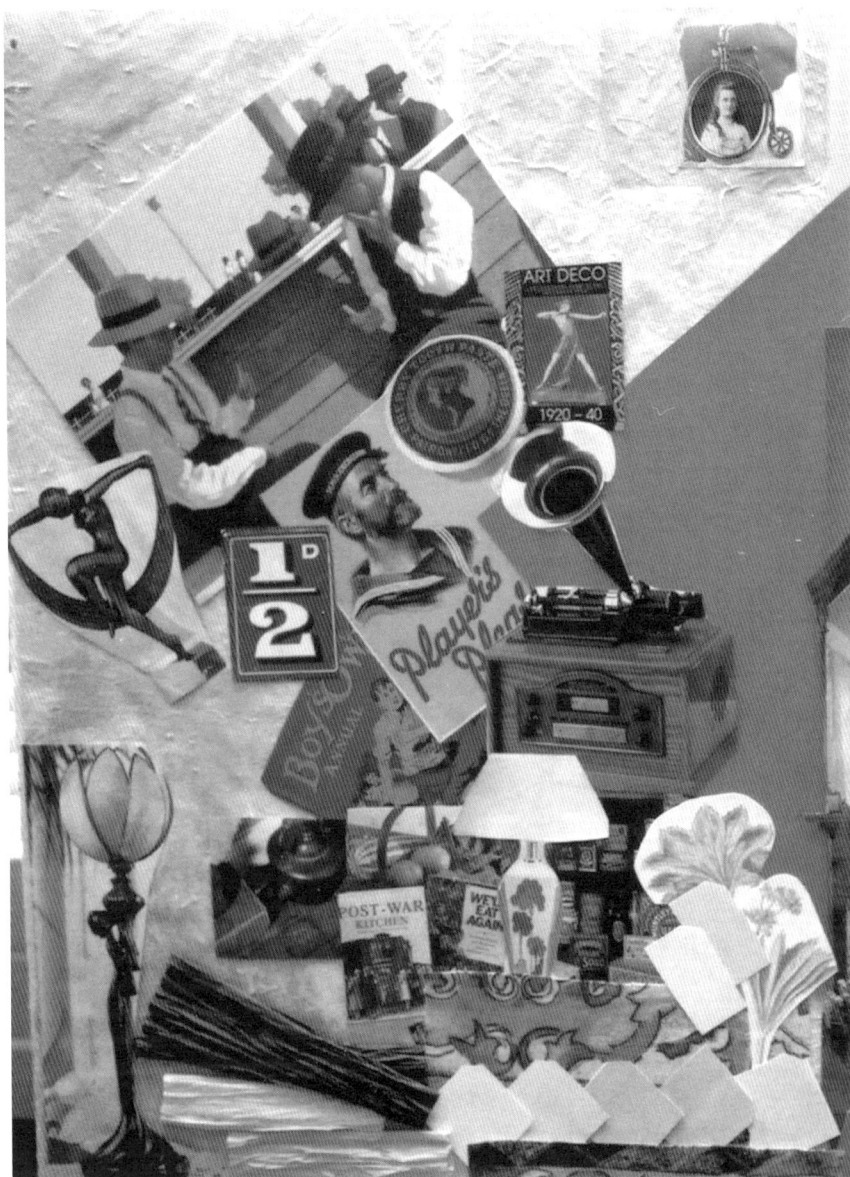

From curtain styles and shades, to pelmets and picture rails, we were soon on the way to having the first coat of paint applied.

We had to obtain permission from the fire officer to paint the doors and unfortunately we were unable to paint or place anything on the main outer door. So our ideas for stained glass soon had to be scrapped. Because of this disappointment we had to find an alternative way of ensuring that people instantly recognised the room for what it was and would feel welcome and encouraged to move on through the main door and into the 1930's/40's front room. I hunted for days to find a wallpaper that simulated brickwork and eventually found the perfect roll. Typical though, it had to be ordered, something my taurean, impatient nature had difficulty coming to terms with. But the wait was well worth it and one evening Lyn, my colleague Jacqui Cridge and I worked late into the evening, cutting out bricks and pasting them to the wall. We intricately positioned a trailing ivy border over the surface, and asked a sign-writer to write the name above the door. I was so pleased with the results; it definitely gave the feeling of someone's front door. The old brown fire door we had been so disappointed with now seemed to pale into insignificance.

We had decided to divide the room up into sections. The kitchen corner, dining area, wartime area, toys and leisure and sitting room with Welsh dresser and fireplace.

But looking around the empty room I began to wish we had called on the services of Anneka Rice. She makes it all seem so easy even if the paint appears not to be dry when they all move in. But there was no Anneka Rice in sight so Fiona was going to have to do, and I used this 'silly' idea to sell my idea to local firms when I went on the scrounge for free paint etc for the room. I always say if you don't ask you don't get and so that's exactly what I did. I phoned Spiller and Webber explaining to them exactly what we were doing and what we were looking for. To my delight the Managing Director very kindly said, "tell me how much paint you want and you can come in and collect it free of charge". Wow! What a result. And Bradfords kindly helped us out in exactly the same way and provided us with all the wood for the picture rails.

Time now to paint and with the help from the talented Mr Mike Stockman, painter and decorator, we turned a set of magnolia walls into three shades of peach, with a dark green picture rail, very authentic and very nice it was too.

Some colour swatches had already been chosen to match perfectly with the wall colour but once again the cost to make curtains and purchase yards and yards of material for the huge bay window all started to seem beyond our reach. I decided to telephone one of my old contacts and friend who worked for Parker Knoll. I had worked with him when I used to sell made to measure chairs as part of my own company The Making Life Easier Centre. Friends can be brilliant contacts and he proved himself to be just that. Not only did Parker Knoll provide us with all the curtain material required but also a wing backed chair. All fire retardant of course which had made the task of finding something authentic just a little harder.

The Welsh dresser proved to be the easiest to convert. We sanded it down and painted the pine one already in situ in the 'make do' reminiscence centre in the day hospital.

Reclamation yards seemed to be my next port of call in search of the authentic fireplace. Every shape, size, colour and design were available. Some were very shabby, some practically new. All expensive and all with the one main problem that the 'guts' of the fire jutted out too far at the back and prevented us from pushing the mantle piece flush against the wall. Not wishing to be beaten by this we continued to scour building sites, antique shops, fire place centres. Finally, one Sunday afternoon my husband came across an identical replica in, believe it or not, the Argos catalogue.

An identical design, but an electric version. Yuck, I hear you all cry. Fair enough it was not the genuine article nor was it scratched or soot ridden, but this would not deter any self respecting occupational therapist to set about distressing and transforming it. And at least it would give that beautiful flickering flame in the corner of the room and give the feeling of warmth and cosiness. Order it, I did and soon after the relevant electrician's checks and the recruiting of two burly men, we had our second main structure in the room. Optimistic as ever I really felt we were getting somewhere.

Another boost came from the Wellington Weekly entitled "Memories are made of music and mothballs". This time I said, "It's all coming together", and so it was. It really was starting to become very exciting. I had stated in the paper also that there would be an authentic fireplace, well a little artistic licence was required here and I also said that authentic metal signs would adorn the front of the building. Whoops! We had all good intentions of carrying this out with signs we had kindly been donated. However we soon changed our minds when we realised the value of them and we felt it would only be tempting fate to place them on the outside of the centre. So as an alternative we employed an artist to paint four replica advertisement signs.

A multi-sensory experience. That was what we were trying to achieve and when visiting the ideal home exhibition I came across a stand selling replica furniture similar to the old doctors' dispensing cabinets with lots of old drawers. They were all made from reclaimed wood, so I ordered one and requested urgent delivery. I told them it was a hospital and so it could be delivered day or night, not really thinking they would take me at my word. So they delivered it at 1 o'clock in the morning and frightened the living daylights out of the night staff. The residential staff were by now beginning to wonder what on earth I was really creating.

The beautiful cabinet had been delivered into the day hospital and it was very heavy to move. Someone who shall remain nameless decided to remove all the drawers and move it into the reminiscence centre, thinking it would lighten the load and make things easier. Three days later, when I think every member of staff, their families and friends had tried but failed abysmally to put all the drawers back in the correct place we were no further on. Of course what we had forgotten was that it was all handmade and each drawer had been made to fit each space perfectly. But not anymore. Final attempt and my son Peter spent a whole afternoon logically trying to remove and replace each drawer in turn but it was no good we would definitely not get out of the room in time to win the crystal! So to this day the drawers are all higgledy piggledy. They are now all full of things to stimulate one's senses, like lavender and rose petals, Brylcream and mothballs, coffee beans and sunlight soap, 4711 and mansion polish. It is a real sensory experience and one not to be missed.

Age Exchange had very kindly told me that I could come and look around their attic store. A place oozing with boxes of items donated to them but of which they had either duplicates or had no immediate use for.

I convinced my long suffering husband Ken who was eating, sleeping and breathing reminiscence, that he would like to drive our company van from DMA Stairlifts to London to collect a few boxes including possibly a kitchen cabinet. I can only describe myself like a child in a toyshop who had just won the lottery. Pam Schweitzer who was the founder of Age Exchange and the instigator for reminiscence in this country said to me, "You may take whatever you want on a long term loan". Help, my brain could not absorb this kind of generosity. I felt giddy with excitement, giggly with nerves and cautious not to appear to be too greedy as I was frantically stuffing things in boxes and making appropriate noises like 'ooh' and 'wow' and 'Oh my goodness', when I came across an even more exhilarating object. It was an absolutely thrilling experience and Ken and I could not stop talking about it on the journey home in the van. How small

minded can one be to be jumping up and down over an old wooden ironing board, or being absolutely spell bound by the tacky tarnished yellow kitchen cabinet with squeaky hinges that would put anyone's fillings on edge. Yet they were all so beautiful in their own way and the things that would put life and real meaning into this room of memories.

So now we had a kitchen area with all the pots and pans, wash-boards and bread bins we required. By the way, Age Exchange had 400 mincers in their store. I'm sure there must be an alternative use for such a popular item for something the public are so readily keen to donate to worthy causes.

A sitting room area with armchairs, sooted up fireplace and rusty old fire-guard with coalscuttle and statutory companion set, a must. A mantle piece strewn with knick knacks and old coins, diggers tobacco and a

charming old clock that used to sit on my Great Auntie Dorothy's own mantle piece. It still ticks in the same old way I remember when I was a child.

The numerous drawers drenched with familiar smells. The taped window and the blackout curtain and the fascinating dug out diaries compiled by my dad and his parents (Granny and Gaffer). Over 1000 entries recording every time they went into the air raid shelter. Graphically describing every last detail. A most fascinating read and one that delivers humility and pulls you up sharply by your senses.

Displayed are tin helmets and ARP badges, stirrup pumps and records / stories of evacuees. This corner, although it may provoke sadness in some will evoke pride and the true British spirit in others.

LOG BOOK OF AIR RAIDS
1940

27

DUG OUT
DRAWING,
NOTE,
ETC:
BOOK.

CANCELLED

28 FEB 1940
28 FEB 1940
28 FEB 1940
28 FEB 1940
28 FEB 1940
28 FEB 1940

AIR RAIDS.

WAR DECLARED
1940 SUNDAY September 3rd
11.0 AM.

~~Monday 2~~
Tuesday 25th June. 1.0 A.M. to 4 A.M. No particular events.

except 1 german plane over High Street Northwood.
3 hours ✓

Thursday Aug 15th 7-10 pm to 7.30 pm. local No incidents

Raid on Croydon

Mrs Mould, Brian haw, Mr + Mrs Lynton, Jill, Elsa, Arthur

180 german aircraft shot down during day

Friday. Aug 16th 12-20 pm to 1-10 pm.

No incidents

Mrs Lynton, Jill, Mr King. Elsa Thames Estuary & S.E. dist.

Friday Aug 16th 5.07 pm to 6-10 pm.

Gunfire heard at 5 pm
No incidents
Raid on Malden Surrey + S.W. Suburbs. Also Herts Bucks & Oxfordshire.

Mrs Lynton, Jill, Elsa.

Sunday Aug 18th 1-10 pm to 2-10 pm

No Incidents

Mr and Mrs Lynton, Jill, Elsa + Arthur

Gunfire heard at 4 pm
E. A. + J away

5-50 to 6-20 pm.

Mrs Lynton + Jill, Mrs Lewey.

Monday. Aug 26ᵗ   3·25 pm to 4 pm   (13)

Mrs Mould, Mrs Lynton
Elsa Arthur + Jim .   Enemy driven off over Thames
      Tea in the dugout.   Eastway.

                                9·30 pm to 315 am.   (14)

Mrs Lynton + Jill, Arthur, Elsa, Jim

All slept in dugout till 3·15.

                        Enemy aircraft continually passed
                        overhead & Heard 8-10 Bombs
                        Some miles away. Also gunfire and
                        Shell bursts towards Uxbridge.

───

Tuesday. Aug 27ᵗʰ   9·30 pm to 12·5 am   (15)
Una, Arthur & Jim   12·30 am to 1·5 am.   (16)

    A. made bunk for Jimmie
    to sleep on in dugout. Very   11·40 p·m   Eight
    successful.   Bombs along
    Slept on till 6·45 am.   East overdown

                                                                45

Friday Sept 13ᵗ.

Arthur, Elsa & Jim had breakfast
in dug out. Elsa in the bath when
Sirens sounded!

7·40AM. to 8·40 A.M   66

Elsa alone at home, Jim at school.
Mr. Riddall brought Jim home at 1·30 pm
as everything quiet locally

9·50AM to 2pm.   67

Elsa, Jimmie & Mrs Law had tea
in dug out.

4 pm to 4·20   68

Elsa, Jimmie, & Arthur.

1 HE, 1 oil bomb on shore of
Hamper Mill Lake. approx 10·10pm

9 pm to 5·30 am.   69

Saturday Sept 14ᵗʰ

Elsa, Arthur & Jimmie
Jim had breakfast in house before
warning. Elsa & arthur had theirs
in shelters. Jim late for Miss North.

9·30 am to 9·50 am   70

Elsa Arthur & Jimmie.

11·0 am to 11·15 am   71

"   "   "   " had tea in shelter.

3·60 pm to 4·50 pm   12

"   "   "   " " supper" "

6·30 pm to 7·15 pm   13

"   "   "   "

7·50 pm to 8·50   14
9·35 pm to 9·53   15

31 Days | Moon Sets 4.4 a.m.
19th Week | Moon Rises 4.59 p.m.

MAY, 1941

Sun Rises 5.20
Sun Sets 8.33

8 THURSDAY (128-237)   N°

(see Wednesday night) A little gunfire &   1.15 am – 4.30 am   576
a number of planes.

Started sleeping upstairs, but a number of   11.55 pm – 4.30 am   577
Huns flew over very low & there was some gunfire
cannon gunfire heard soon after we reached shelter where
we all slept rest of night. E saw searchlights & so him bedroom window.
(Chief attacks on Humber district & Midlands.
14 brought down.) St Vincents Hosp this demolished by H.E. Incendiaries
near Roberts farm. Hun brought down & crashed on Ruislip Golf Course. Bombs at
Hemel Hempstead.

9 FRIDAY (129-236)
Half-quarter Day (England)

All slept in our bedroom.
No heavy attacks throughout the country but 3 men brought down.

10 SATURDAY (130-235)
Heavy barrage on
All slept in shelter. Also Mrs Kidd. Guns close at times.   11.01 pm – 5.55 am   578
A very heavy raid on London. Planes almost continuously overhead from about
till dawn, partly our fighters. Machine gun & cannon fire heard. Also bombs
which fell at Harrow & also Denham. Glow seen towards Edgware.
Among places hit were House of Commons, Westminster Abbey, Baker St
station No 4 platform. Met. interrupted beyond Baker St. Other hits on Druces
Pentonville, Theobalds Rd. (this Prison offices damaged again) Queens Hall, Old Bailey
Holborn (1 Rly) station, Cheltenham St, Holborn Viaduct, & City generally
Ludgate Hill

About 5 am a huge billowing cloud of smoke seen N East. Still visible at
four. caused by huge
fire in London.
33 Jerries brought down.   (see above)

47

'4   1.55 am – 2.25 am. {Heard 4 F/8s explode a few   1058
      (distance away.
During afternoon & 1 am away heard many Rockets
exploding at varying distances. 14 in all & chine rather.
Below one was at Hendon.
25/1 About 8.20 am Heard Rocket which exploded in
mid air over Dollis Hill
27/1 About 4 am awakened by Rocket which exploded
in mid air over St anmore. Blast opened bedroom windows
29/1 Roused at 6.20 am by fairly distant Rocket.
1/2 about 3 am extremely sharp Rocket explosion awakened us.
11/2 Very loud Rocket about 5 am. It exploded near Fulmer
15/2 Loudest Rocket yet about 9 am.
17/2 Roused by Rocket about 4.30 am.
                            an Eastcote Sqr
2/3 Saw heard Rocket exploded to the E. about 11.00 hrs. went during night.

3   2.40 hrs – 2.48 hrs. {Heard 3 F/8s anyways & (1st lot of   1059
                (the long narrow bend bone type) 3 wow
                (rather big one explosion.
   4.07 hrs – 4.15 hrs. Heard 1 F/8 E & A at Mill End   1060

4   12.45 am – 1.50 am.   2 F/8's.   1061
           Northwood again about 11 am.
   11.55 am – 12.05 am. One Very loud F/8   1062
     Northwood about 10.50
5   12.29 am — 12.41 am   1 big explosion heard towards Stanmore.   1063

6   11.05 hrs – 11.10 hrs   One F/8 heard   1064
Rockets heard so frequently mass than it
is useless to note down their times. One fell at
corner of Smithfield on 8/3 about 4 am and
another near Hendon on 12.45 am. 9/3

14   9.25 am – 9.31 am {E on duty, went to Post.   1065
                {Heard F/8 followed by explosion.
                {Fell on Ordnance Factory at Cranford
19   8.14 am – 8.25 am   One explosion heard ? F/8   1066

20   9.15 hrs – 9.57   —   1067
Rockets are getting stepped up apparently.
Night 20/21 we were awakened 5 times one was at Stanmore and
another Pinner Hill. About 6 during the day One at Packards
the West Rd. and the London one at 6.40 It fell in the
air 2½ miles away towards Ruislip & another during night of 22/23 am
also E gas burn one which fell at Chignal
and so on and so on

24   7.10 am – 7.20 am   1068
     7.50 am – 8.03 am   1069
25   7.55 am – 8.10 am   Heard one F/8 explode   1070
27   2.45 am – 2.57 am   – " –   1071
28   8.00 am – 8.07 am   – " –   1072
29   9.00 am – 9.07 am   – " –   1073

30   A's last Duty
1-2   J's last Stand By.
2   F's last Duty   And End of Civil Defence.
       May 8th   VE DAY!!!

48

A L E R T S.

MONTH	1939	1940	1941	1942	1943	1944	1945
Jan.	–	0	31	0	5	6	4
Feb.	–	0	34	0	1	14	0
March.	–	0	32	0	4	10	14
April.	–	0	21	0	6	5	0
May.	–	0	11	0	10	1	0
June.	–	1	4	0	6	28	–
July.	–	0	2	5	0	117	–
August.	–	27	2	5	1	127	–
Sept.	3	110	2	2	2	17	–
Oct.	0	111	1	3	13	16	–
Nov.	0	82	1	0	9	7	–
Dec.	0	29	1	0	7	7	–
Annual Total.	3	360	142	15	64	349	18
Grand Total.	3	363	505	520	584	933	951

MONTHLY DURATION OF ALERTS.

MONTH	1939	1940	1941	1942	1943	1944	1945
Jan.	–	0	2d8h49m	0	3h.29m	5h15m	1h13m
Feb.	–	0	1d19h17m	0	20m	10h47m	0
March.	–	0	1d23h29m	0	2h.54m	7h58m	4h46m
Apl.	–	0	1d22h53m	0	3h.54m	2h42m	0
May.	–	0	1d.3h46m	0	4h.55m	42m	0
June.	–	2h.52m.	8h.58m	0	1h.47m	2d2h55m	–
July.	–	0	2h.26m	6h.25m.	0	4d22h19m	–
Aug.	–	1d15h46m	1h.4m.	1h.49m	53m	2d15h53m	–
Sept.	2hr49m.	11d14h6m	2h.12m	59m	45m	7h37m	–
Oct.	0	11d11h5m	1h.18m	33m	7h.55m	4h28m	–
Nov.	0	10d6h23m	1h.5m.	0	4h.1m	2h18m	–
Dec.	0	3d15h44m	26m.	0	3h.48m	3h24m	–
Annual Total	2h.49m	38d18h47m	9d23h43m	9h.46m	1d10h41m	11d14h28m	5h59m
Grand Total.	2h.49m	38d21h36m	48d21h19m	49d7h5m	50d17h46m	62d8h14m	62d14h13m

LONGEST ALERT IN EACH MONTH.

MONTH	1939	1940	1941	1942	1943	1944	1945
Jan.	–	0	4h 33m	0	1h 28m	1h 23m	30m
Feb.	–	0	4h 11m	0	29m	1h 11m	0
March.	–	0	6h 2m	0	1h 31m	1h 33m	1h12m
April.	–	0	7h 37m	0	1h 3m	59m	0
May.	–	0	6h 14m	0	55m	42m	0
June.	–	0	4h 1m	0	35m	9h 47m	–
July.	–	2h 52m	2h 11m	2h 19m	0	8h 7m	–
Aug.	–	0	37m	28m	53m	5h 49m	–
Sept.	2h 14m	7h 1m	1h 58m	46m	38m	1h 17m	–
Oct.	0	10h 15m	1h 18m	14m	1h 47m	40m	–
Nov.	0	13h 38m	1h 5m	0	52m	47m	–
Dec.	0	13h 47m	26m	0	53m	44m	–

Bombs exclusive of 1 Kg 1 Bs.   Casualities.   Houses.

Shells	38	Fatal	7	Destroyed	31
Bombs & Mines	94	Slight & Serious	80	Seriously damaged	135
Flybombs	1	Injured by M.G.	1	Slightly "	1250
Totals	133	Bullet.	88		1416

The highest number of alerts in 24 hours was 9 on 29/7/1944 and 17/8/1944.

49

AIR RAID PRECAUTIONS, RICKMANSWORTH

with

S U M M A R Y

of

AIR RAID ALERTS and

RESULTANT DAMAGE

in

RICKMANSWORTH URBAN DISTRICT COUNCIL
A.R.P. DISTRICT.

during

THE GERMAN WAR

1939 - 1945.

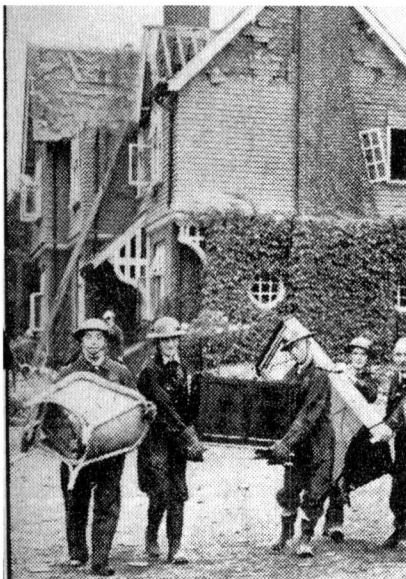

Shop Fronts Blown Out

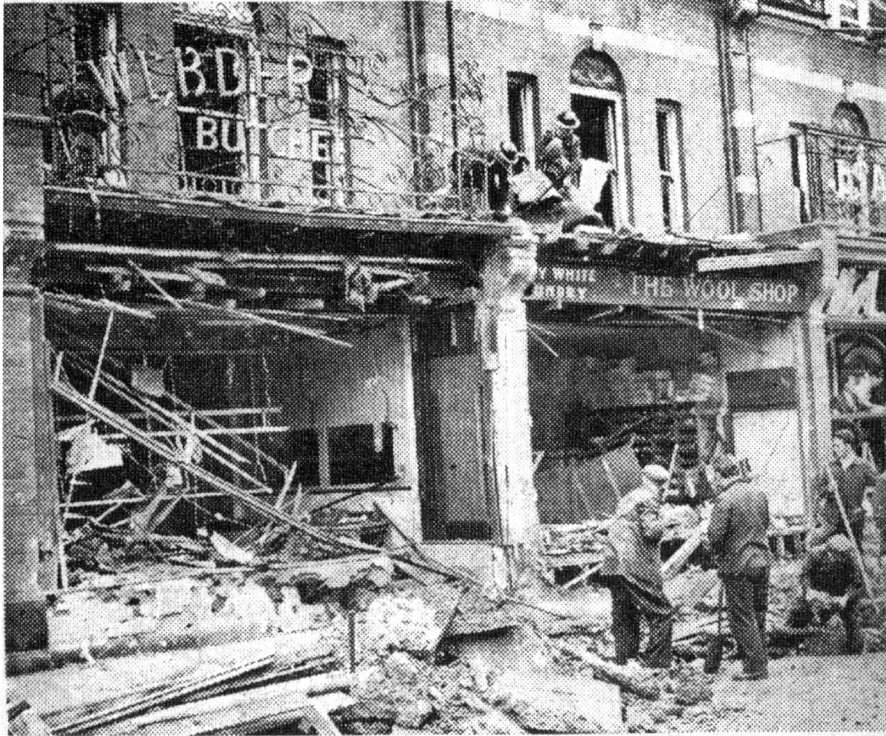

To-day's picture in a London suburb of wreckage after the night raid.

Direct Hit—Boy Unhurt

WED
28 AUG
1940

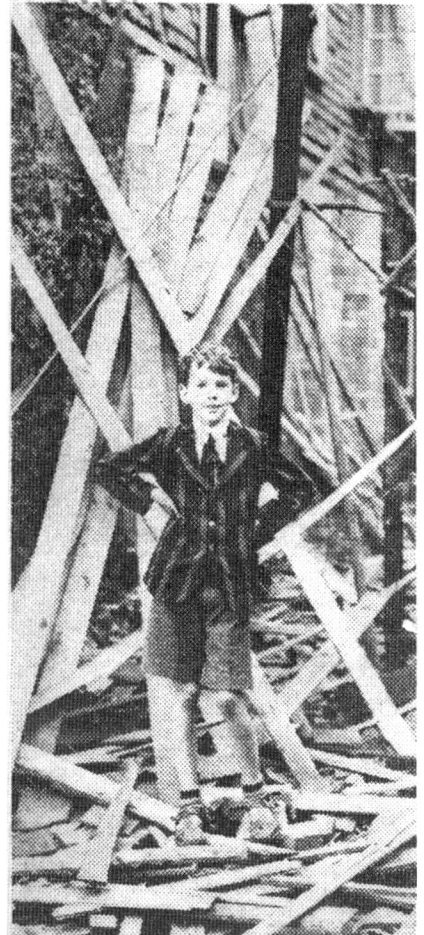

To-day's picture of a lucky boy—Ian Stewart, aged nine, who was unhurt when his house, outside the London area, was hit by a bomb in last night's raid. He and the maid were alone in the house. His parents were away.

51

Mr Perry, a war enthusiast, kindly donated a gas mask perfectly preserved in its original cardboard box. Although we are unable to allow people to try it on, it is a curt reminder to many of the anxiety and fear many experienced during the war years.

Many local people on hearing about the room dug deep into their possessions at home and came up to the day hospital clutching precious memorabilia they wanted to donate. We made an agreement from the beginning that nothing from outsiders would be on loan . A form was created and individuals signed to say that it had been permanently donated to the centre (see appendix 1).We felt this would save any embarrassment or awkward situations in the future and it was sound advice we had taken from Age Exchange.

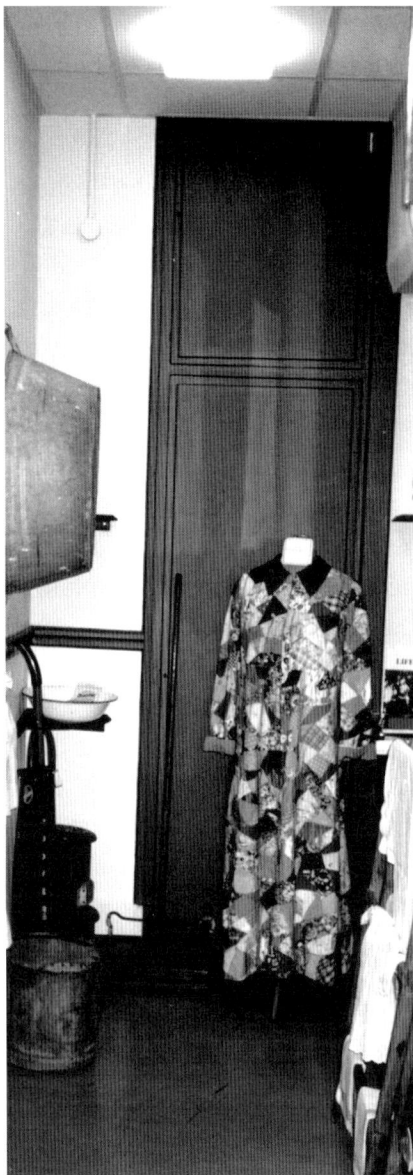

A very touching donation came from a lady who had a dressing gown that reminded me of Joseph's coat of many colours. It had been made out of patchwork and the material came from all the party dresses she had had as a child. She seemed to be proud to hand it over and pleased we gave it pride of place in the corridor area outside the main room.

A treadle sewing machine donated by Pyrland House became the main focus in the leisure area. Surrounding this a selection of silver plated picnic sets, ice skates with leather boots attached and my Gran's old lace pillow and beautifully carved bobbins. Unfortunately the pillow had been tampered with whilst in the other temporary area and some of the bobbins had been detached and the threads tangled, but it still had fond memories for me as my son's christening robe that proudly hangs in my own wardrobe at home was made on this very pillow.

Toys spill out of an old toy box and a school desk scrawled with graffiti holding old school books and slates. A pair of conkers lay tangled together in the bottom and the shove ha'penny board scratched and well worn sat with a lonely coin ready to be played. The John Bull printing set with those funny little rubber letters and the tweezers. A big old hand-made red train engine that had belonged to my dad lay on the floor. It definitely would not have passed any health and safety test today.

All the collection of antiquities and trinkets collected from Gaffer's garage and house and all the finery from Age Exchange were gathered together and scattered amongst the furniture and themed areas. My Gran's wedding dress and the smoking jacket belonging to Gaffer were hung up with a picture of them on their wedding day featured below. The photographer enlarged and framed my relatives pictures and the ribbon plates, iron bath, resource material and shelves for the sweet jars and china were all carefully screwed to the wall with precision. You could now stand in front of the mantle piece and admire yourself in the oval mirror precariously suspended by a chain, or fish into one of the drawers to feel a real silk stocking or delve into the oak medicine cabinet made by my husband in 1954 to discover the snow fire and ridged glass bottles and those old fashioned smells. I wanted this room to be a place where everybody could share their memories, where you could sit quietly and reflect on the good old days or pick up a 1938 newspaper and re-live the moment. The gramophone and wireless donated by Philip Knighton from the shop in Wellington could provide the resonant tones of Glen Miller or Vera Lynn.

As I sat there in the room in the same place that I had first had this spectacular idea I reminisced about how it all began and how far we had now come. My dream certainly had become reality. There were so many things that had happened along the way and so many stories to be told. It truly was great fun and as I sat reflecting, I looked at all the artefacts that bestowed this wondrous room and thought to myself, if only they could speak for themselves what a marvellous collection of tales we would have to share.

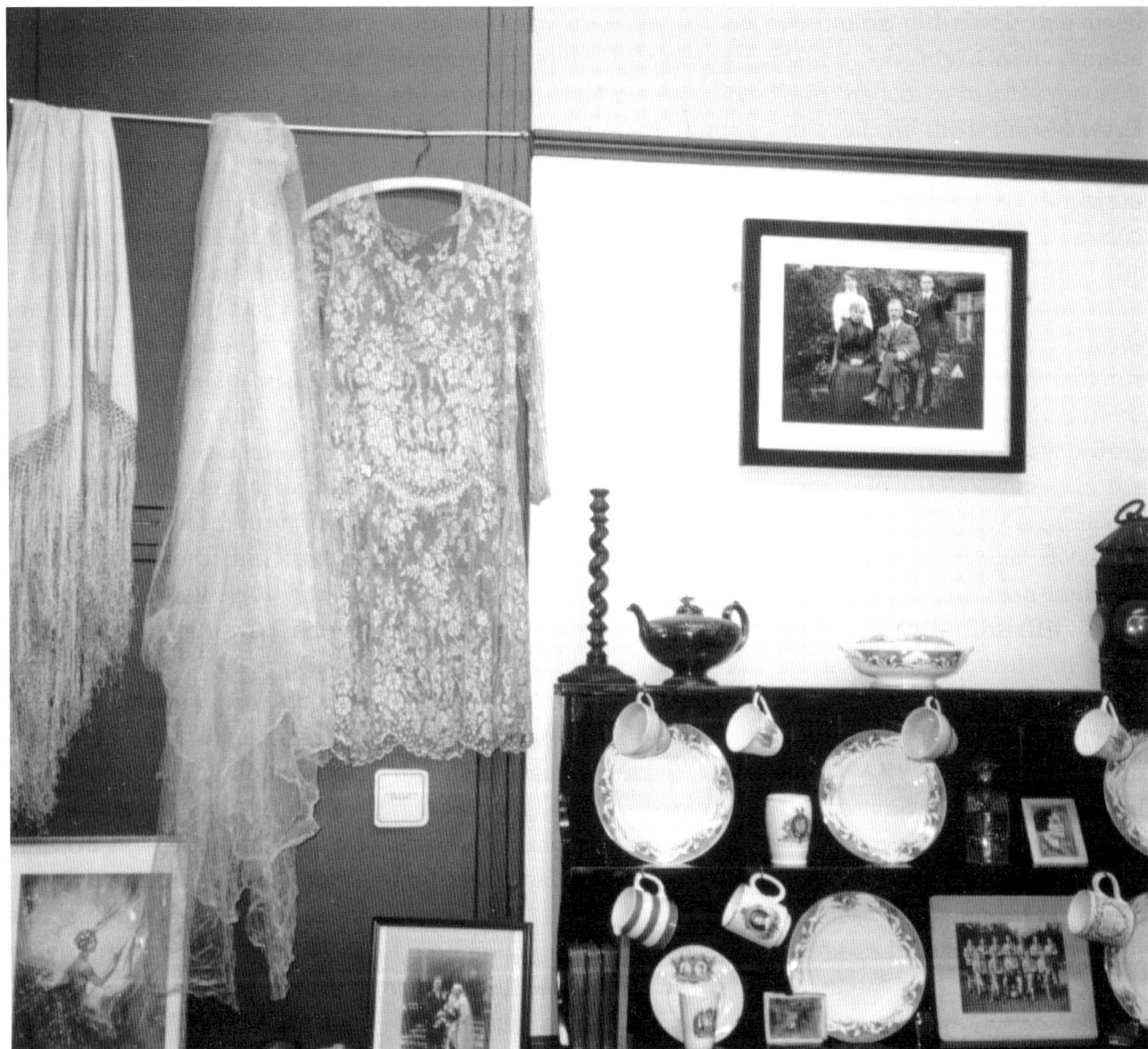

54

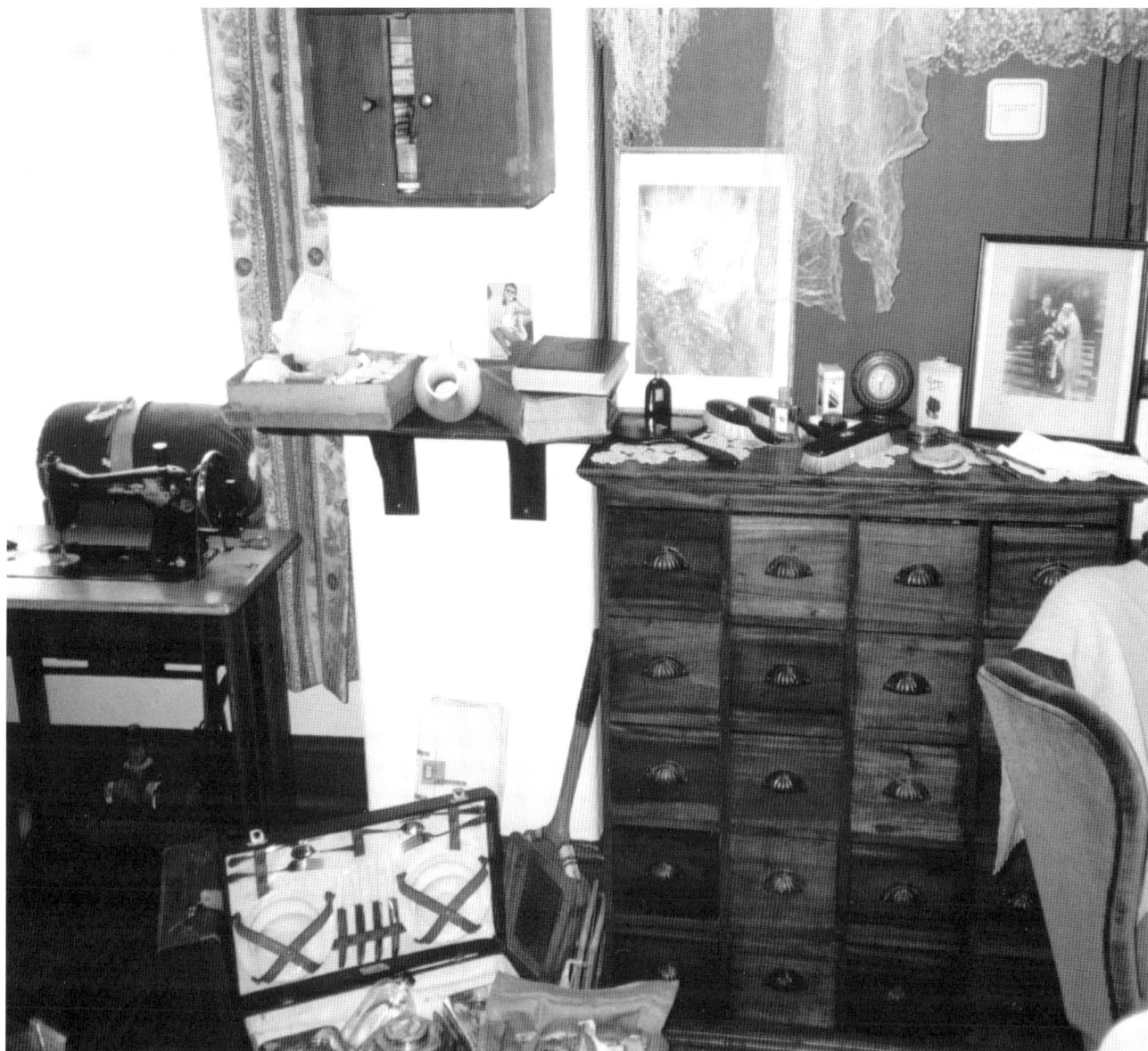

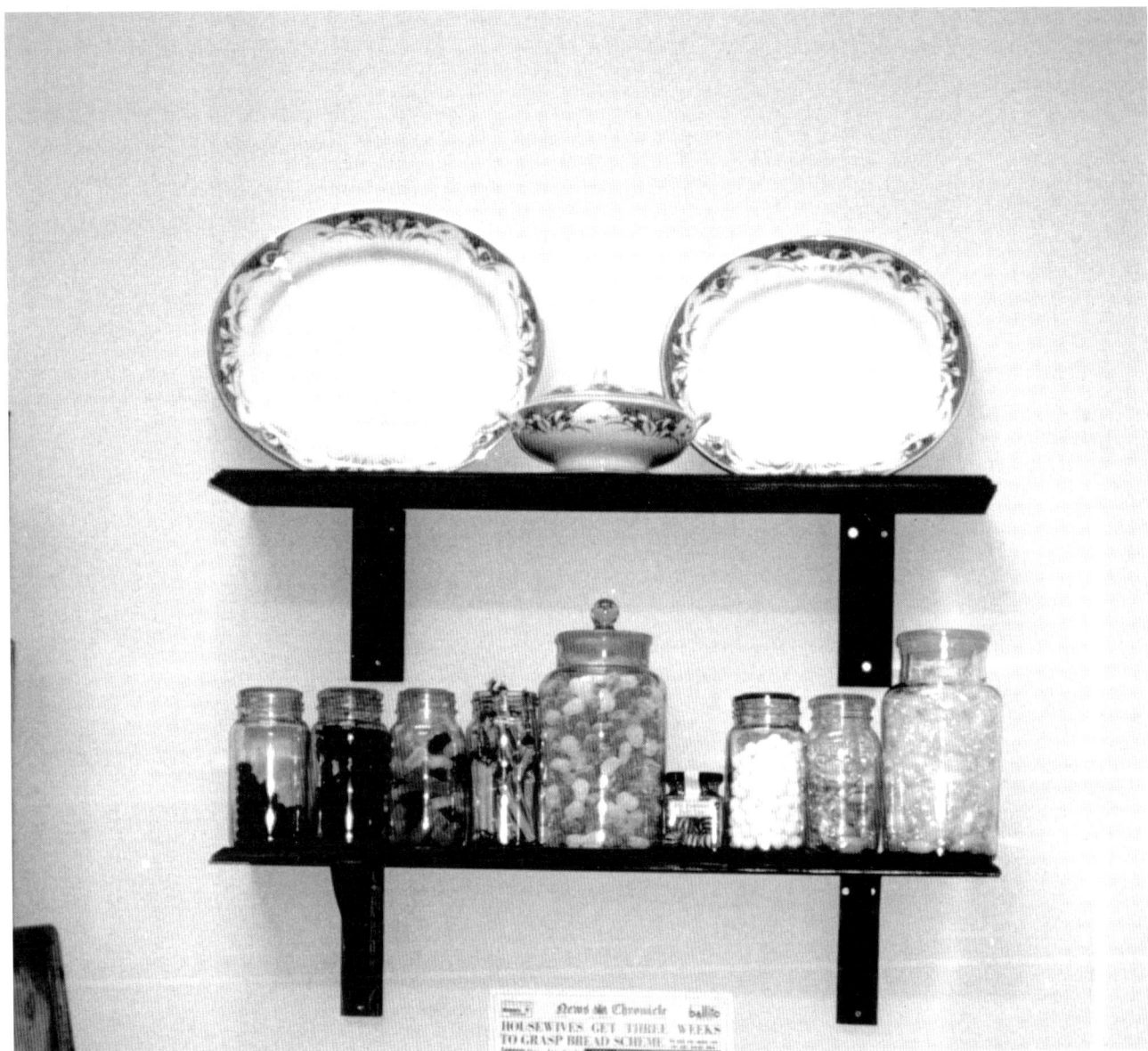

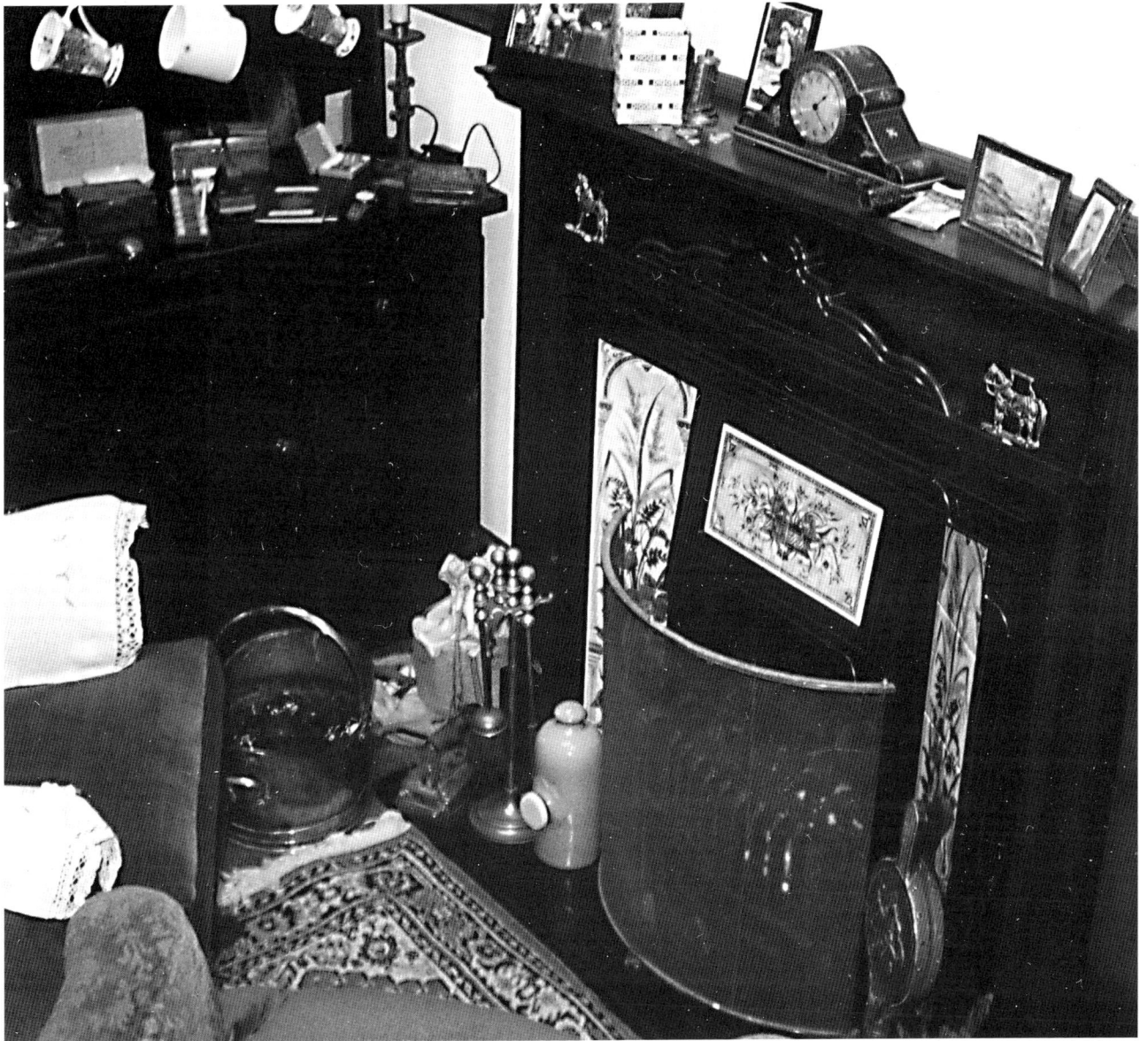

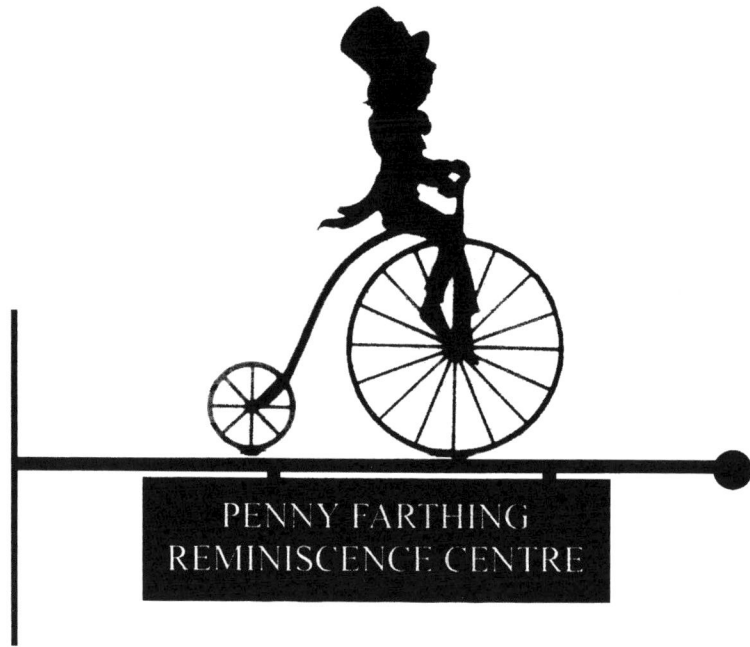

PENNY FARTHING
REMINISCENCE CENTRE

4. Time to celebrate

Tuesday 6th July 1998 and the article in the Wellington Weekly reads as follows: " An old fashioned 1940's style street party, complete with gramophone music from the era, is being planned to celebrate the opening of Wellington's Penny Farthing Reminiscence Centre".

Yes, we had at last decided on a name and having toyed with naming it "Goodnight Sweetheart" after the television series starring Nicholas Lyndhurst, "Second Time Around" and "All our Yesterdays" we finally chose Ken's idea, "The Penny Farthing Reminiscence Centre". We realised that it was out of date but we needed a name that instantly conjured up somewhere old and would not be mixed up with something 'saucy' or a second hand clothes shop. So Penny Farthing it became.

A day hospital trip to the flower show in Vivary Park very nicely provided a sign. We could not believe our eyes when the Otter Signs stand, selling mainly weathervanes, actually had artwork depicting a penny-farthing. It was obviously meant to be.

I had originally got the idea of having a miniature penny-farthing displayed outside when I saw a bright yellow one hanging above the King's Cycle shop in Station Road. I even went as far as to ring them to see if they had a contact. But they explained that they had bought it years ago in a junk shop and painted it to fit in with their company image.

Of course any one who comes from Taunton would know that Spiller and Webber own a life size and genuine penny farthing, used for their publicity, so of course we had to cajole them into lending it to us for our street party opening. They were more than open to the suggestion but it would have to be on a day when the delivery man worked. This started to dictate the day and date of the opening day and therefore required a little re-thinking. But we could not miss a chance like this. So move the date that actually seemed originally to be so flexible, it was wavering in the wind like an out of control kite. So what's different! We would now have to tether down these ideas and make some firm arrangements, after all we had now had a piece in the Wellington Weekly and they said it was set to open the last week in August by "VERA LYNN". Who's mad idea was that? No prizes for guessing!!!

Nicholas Lyndhurst had actually been the first agent I contacted through Artist Index in London. Finally after numerous phone calls I managed to speak to him, the agent that is, not Nicholas himself but our request was unsuccessful.

Artist Index could not seem to produce any alternative names of possible artists and so it was back to the drawing board.

What about an old Wellington School boy? Perhaps David Suchet, as Hercule Poirot?

There were many other names who were lawyers and very successful businessmen

GLENDA JACKSON, M.P.

HOUSE OF COMMONS
LONDON SW1A 0AA

Fiona Mahoney
Senior Occupational Therapist   0171-219 4008
Somerset Partnership NHS and Social Care Trust
Stratfield House
Bulford
Wellington
Somerset TA21 8QQ

10 June 1999

Dear Ms Mahoney

Thank you for your recent invitation to open the 'Penny Farthing' Reminiscence Centre.

I am afraid that, due to the pressure of Ministerial and Constituency duties, I will not be able to come. But I would like to send you my very best wishes for your imaginative project which will I am sure be of great benefit to the whole community.

Yours sincerely

GLENDA JACKSON MP

House of Commons

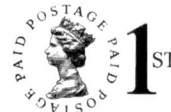

POSTAGE PAID POSTAGE PAID 1ST

but nobody that sprung to mind as recognisable or an appropriate celebrity.

I had hoped Age Exchange might be able to help. Perhaps they had a patron? Yes they did Glenda Jackson. But no joy, she sent a very polite reply from the House of Commons stating that due to the pressure of Ministerial and Constituency duties she would be unable to attend.

So Dame Vera Lynn had to be our next port of call. Her Agency is called Angel and I was hoping that my Guardian Angel was looking down on me, but she obviously was busy looking down on someone less fortunate than myself. Vera very kindly sent me a hand written letter of regret, but none the less the letter has become a very treasured possession, that takes pride of place in the photographic archive.

Dame Vera Lynn, D.B.E., LL.D., M.Mus.

Dear Fiona Mahoney,

Thank you for your letter, I am very sorry, but owing to so many commitments in my diary. I shall not be able to be with you on the week of the 24 August.

I hope you have a successful week and the weather is kind to you.

Best Wishes to all

Yours

Vera Lynn

So feeling quite bereft we decided to be slightly less ambitious and use someone closer to home. We approached one of our own talented television celebrities, Clive Gunnell, a West Country television presenter. We actually could not believe our good luck and fortune when he said yes. The date of the Street Party opening could finally be set and the final arrangements could at last begin. We were now running approximately one month late, but not to worry. We needed to put together an invitation and Sue Rapsey (a colleague), kindly made a pencil sketch of a penny-farthing with a fantastic old lamppost, one of which I had fallen in love with on my trips around the reclamation sites but to date is still not in situ outside the reminiscence room. A little more fund raising required I think!

Wellington Weekly under the headline, 'Pioneering Centre's day to remember', reported that we intended to have a "grand" knees-up. "A street party with trestle tables, bunting, flags, music and dancing is planned. Vintage cars, buses and a genuine penny-farthing will all be on display with patients, staff and members of the NHS Trust as well as locals dressed in costumes".

Well after hours stuffing and licking endless amounts of envelopes, writing press releases and posting what seemed to be hundreds of invitations, not forgetting the sleepless nights, the day of reckoning was finally upon us.

We had spent many treatment sessions in the day hospital working through the numerous topics and subjects surrounding the 1930's and 40's and everyone had spent weeks searching deep in

PENNY FARTHING
REMINISCENCE
CENTRE

Take a trip down memory lane, by visiting Wellington's new and exciting attraction.

A place where memories of the 30's and 40's are brought to life.

***

The centre is made up of a variety of areas, including:

- Fire place with hearth and mantlepiece
- War time corner
- Leisure & music
- Multi-sensory environment

Together with lots of artifacts & memorabilia.

There is also a place to sit, with a cup of tea and browse through old books, or just sit and recall the past.

***

The centre will be officially opened at 2.30 pm by:

CLIVE GUNNELL
West Country TV Presenter

on

Thursday 30th September 1999

***

The centre will offer regular reminiscence sessions, which will be open to everyone. Details of these are attached.

***

Any artifacts or memorabilia of the era (30's & 40's) are still being gathered together and would be gratefully received.

For more details contact:

Fiona Mahoney
on
01823 661663

Stratfield House, Wellington & District Cottage Hospital, Bulford, Wellington, Somerset, TA21 8QQ

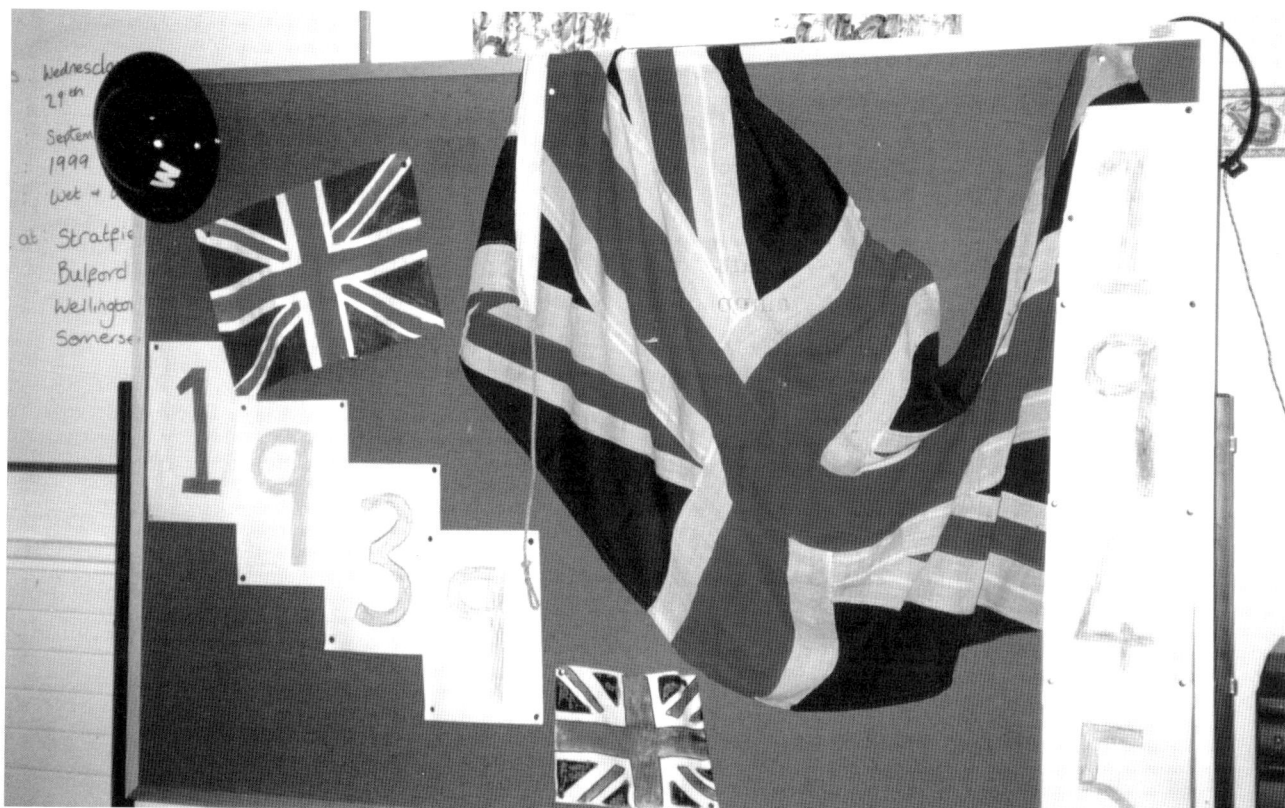

trunks and lofts at home to uncover that well loved wrap-around apron or once worn old warden's helmet that they were sure they had kept for a moment just like this. Unfortunately it seemed that many a jumble sale or charity shop had been the lucky recipient of these now most wanted and longed for items. We tried fancy dress shops and local newspapers begging for items of clothing but it seems we definitely live in a throw away world. My colleagues and friends probably would tell you that I am a bit of a hoarder, but this lack of costumes has just reinforced the need to hoard even more. A panic phone call to Age Exchange in London and more begging proved to be successful and although we were only days away from September 30th I was

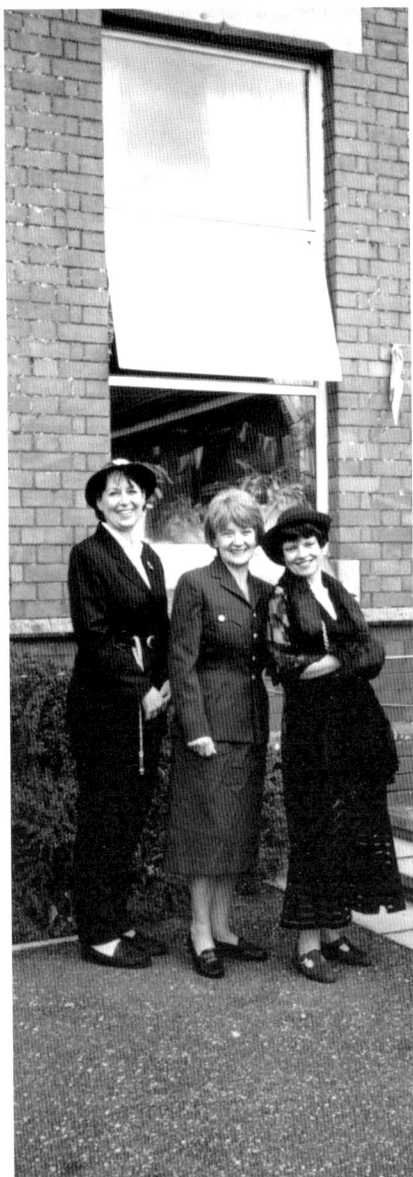

reassured that the costumes we had requested e.g. anything they could spare, would be with us before 2.00pm on the opening day. Note this was the opening time.

A final late night clean up in the reminiscence centre, and the morning arrived. Everyone seemed to be scurrying around like ants, as though some child had just stuck a stick into their nest. There just seemed to be so much to do. And believe it or not the costumes still had not arrived. Suddenly everyone that had been patiently awaiting the additional costumes had to become an air raid warden only because the fancy dress shop had a surplus of hats following the VE day celebrations.

Bunting was strewn from building to building, flags draped and nailed to walls.

The trestle tables were

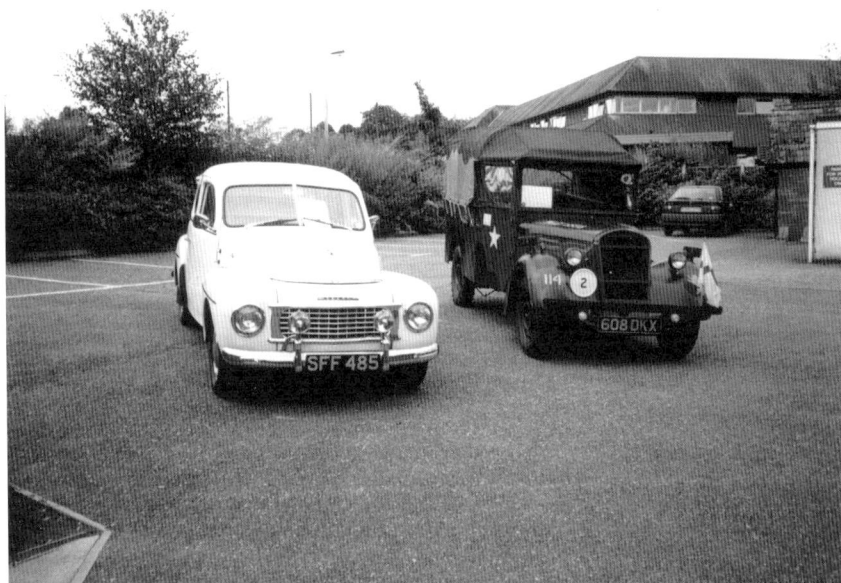

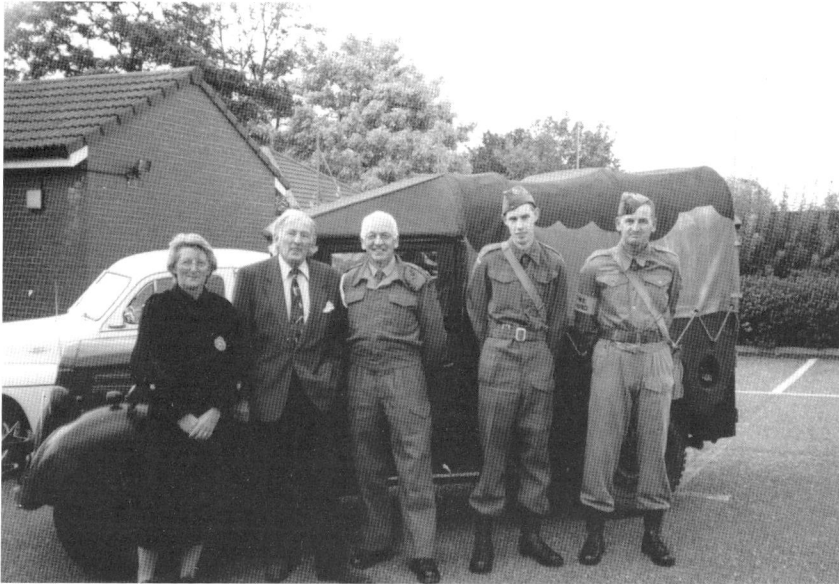

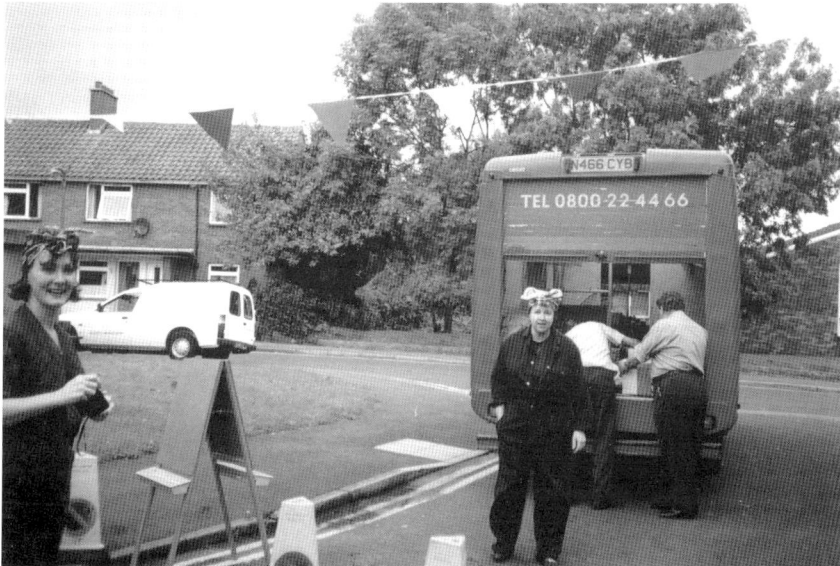

erected and the vintage cars and army jeeps shown to their parking places.

The large van housing the genuine penny-farthing reversed into the grounds and off loaded the splendid bike. Tables lay with sandwiches, made of spam and jam, cakes and scones.

1.30pm and the best sight of the day, was when the red Post Office van pulled in and delivered two boxes of costumes. Frantically we opened the boxes and pulled out costume after costume. Those who had been promised something to wear but had made do were now stripping off items to change into something different, rushing to the mirror to glance at the new look. Headscarves were tied, aprons adjusted, trousers changed for skirts and Army men became Naval officers. It was complete and utter pandemonium and those

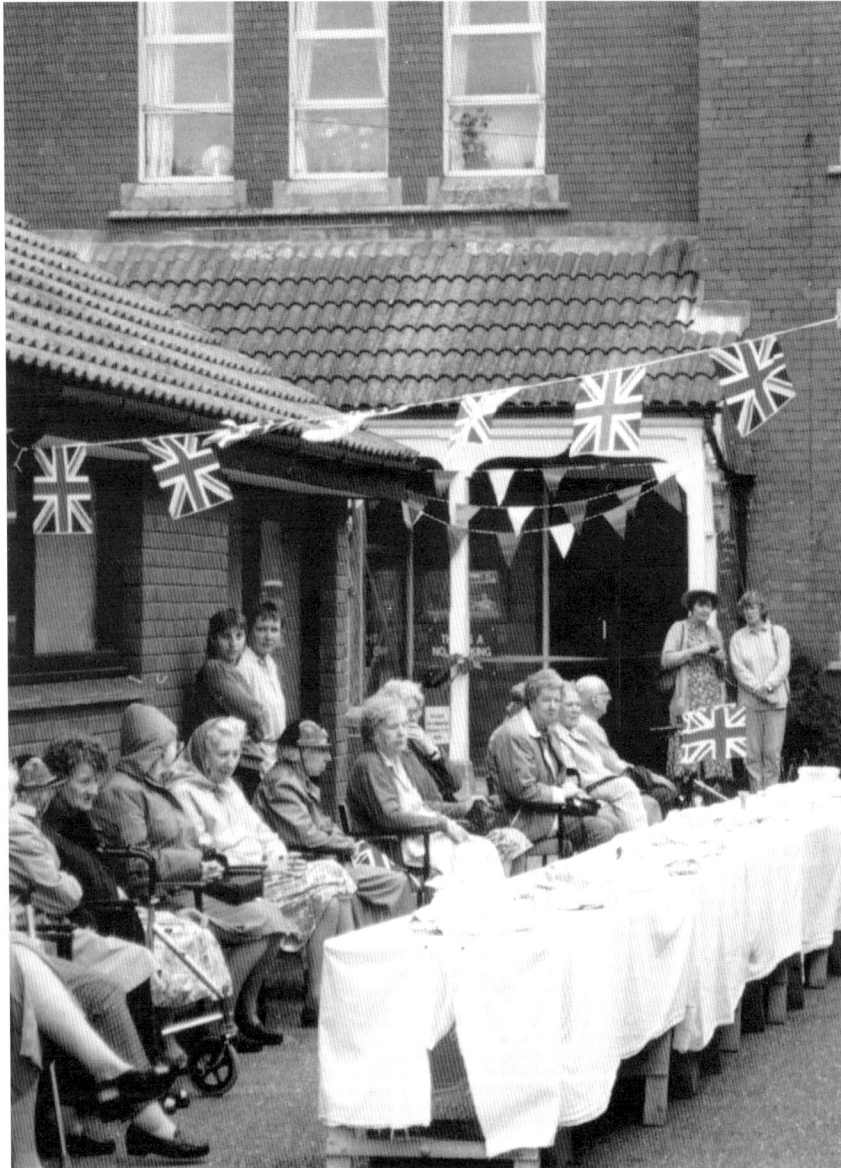

precious minutes were quickly ticking away.

Clive Gunnell had just appeared and announced that unfortunately his wife Hilary Bonner was unwell and so he was alone. Another slight change as we were planning to present a bouquet of flowers to his wife, but never mind we would have to present them to Clive instead. A scene that actually seemed slightly strange and unusual at the time.

Well Vera Lynn may not have been there in person but her music was ringing all around us.

Everyone sat around the trestle tables and awaited the opening ceremony. The ribbon tied across the doors of the Wellington Cottage Hospital and entrance to the new Penny Farthing Reminiscence Centre was finally cut. My vision had at last become reality.

Rain stopped play approximately ten minutes after the speeches and everyone hurriedly bustled and jostled their way into the day hospital where a contingency plan was then set in motion (due to the recent gloomy weather forecast) and a second street party had been laid up with the appropriate bunting, flags etc.

For a brief moment I stepped back to listen, watch and absorb the atmosphere. Everyone seemed to be smiling and laughing and of course reminiscing. I could feel my heart swollen with pride. I had an overwhelming sense of achievement and the satisfaction that now others could share in my dream.

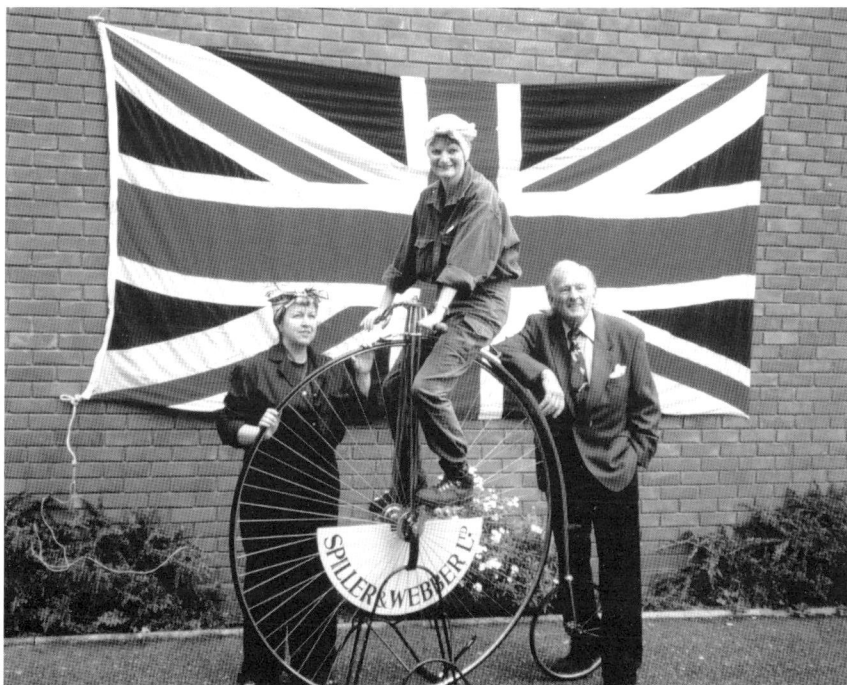

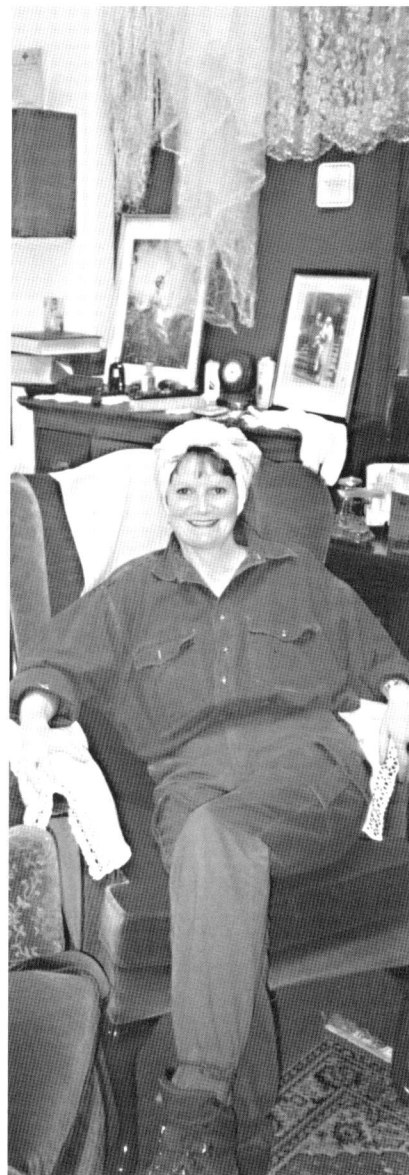

5. The way ahead

So at last we are there. A room full of other people's memories and treasures, bulging with history and every piece with a story to tell all of its own. My original aim had been to set this room up for anyone and every one to use but I think if I'm honest the easy bit was now over and the real hard work had begun to ensure it was used to its best and fullest extent. We had already planned a timetable with pre-booked sessions for the local community and schools but mainly for use by Stratfield House. We allocated themed sessions for Stratfield covering musical appreciation, sensory awareness, use of the boxes and specific themes plus looking back at newspapers.

The League of Friends had kindly agreed to staff the community afternoon and we hoped that the day centres and residential homes would also make use of it.

All the sessions would need to be pre-booked to prevent them being interrupted and to ensure someone was there to open up, introduce people to the room and explain how to use it and most importantly ensure that the lights and fire had been turned off and the room locked securely afterwards. This was something that actually proved to be quite a time-consuming problem, especially if I wasn't there. My colleague Jacqui Cridge was a tower of strength. She had already spent many a long evening with me in the reminiscence centre, displaying, cleaning, arranging and generally being a brilliant moral support. She began to take on more and more responsibility for the centre and was always there to help me out when I was unable to open up for whatever reason.

A leaflet was soon put together to aid this dilemma entitled "How to use the reminiscence room" (see chapter 6). A document that saved a great deal of time and allowed people something to take away as well as provide an explanation of why this room had been created and its intentions for use.

We also ensured we had written and displayed a disclaimer on the wall of the centre partly because some of

TIMETABLE - PENNY FARTHING REMINISCENCE ROOM

	MONDAY	TUESDAY	WEDNESDAY	THURSDAY	FRIDAY
AM **10.30 - 12.00**	Stratfield House Musical Appreciation Morning	Stratfield House Sensory Awareness Morning	Pre-booked Sessions for Local Schools	Stratfield House Residential Group	Pre-booked Sessions for Day Centre/ Residential Homes/ Hosptial Units
PM **1.30 - 3.00**	Pre-booked Session for Day Centre/ Residential Homes/ Hospital Units	Open Community Afternoon Supervised by Volunteers	Stratfield House Theme Group or Looking Back @ Newspaper Cuttings	Stratfield House Individual Reminiscence Group	Stratfield House Sensory/Music Awareness

the older items were rusty or had sharp edges and did not comply with today's rigorous health and safety standards. We did not want anyone to hurt themselves and so this notice just put out a warning and made people aware. (see appendix 2)

We created a comprehensive reference area in the corridor outside the room comprising of videos and books with fascinating titles such as "A Somerset Christmas", "Tomorrow's Antiques", "Winter Warmers", "Yesterday's Shopping", "The 20th Century" "The Lost Street", "The Morcombe and Wise Show".

Promotion, publicity and marketing suddenly became the buzz -words I found myself using. I realised that in order for this centre to be successful people had to know of its existence. Obviously I had many stoic supporters along the way who had trusted my judgement, consoled my fears, bounced along with my enthusiasm and shared the drive, motivation and determination that I exuded. But was that enough? If my intoxication and passion waned would they all be there, flying the flag? I feared that they would not and so I had to ensure that the long awaited centre, now completed and up and running was there to stay. The Penny Farthing Centre had to continue to impress and fascinate the whole community and become a permanent feature that would put Wellington on the map. The newspaper continued to serve us well and the editor of the Somerset Partnership Newsletter had kindly given us pride of place on the front page. The phone began to ring and interested parties from around the trust and the local community soon started to book in trips and sessions. We had to keep a diary to prevent double booking and although it was only just a steady, regular flow, of people, not the football crowd I had described to the newspaper earlier at our Christmas Fayre, we could not put ourselves under any additional pressure.

The boxes were also of great interest and we started to hire them out at the reasonable cost of only £10.00 per week. This made the introduction and usage of these reminiscence tools a very viable and cost effective way of delivering reminiscence over a few treatment sessions. It soon became clear that although there was a considerable interest in reminiscence, many felt they were lacking in the knowledge, confidence and competence to facilitate, plan and deliver the reminiscence groups to their clients/ patients.

Following an invitation to an international conference in Stockholm on Reminiscence, I decided with an occupational therapy colleague, Muriel Coles to plan and present a conference entitled "A positive approach to dementia". The conference assisted those with a limited knowledge of reminiscence to increase and improve their abilities and enable them to feel more competent at facilitating reminiscence groups in the future. It also helped to promote awareness of the Penny Farthing Reminiscence Centre.

On 12th October 1999 I am quoted in the paper as saying "In the future I want to use the centre as a building block and add in a computer resource and include maybe a library and museum and get in an art therapist and music and drama therapist to do intergenerational reminiscence between young and old. This is what I would like to achieve eventually".

Well since that date I have created many additional building blocks and have started to build my reminiscence tower of success.

First Building Block

My first building block is the "National and European" block. We were invited by Age Exchange Reminiscence Centre in London to be 1 of 5 in the country piloting a new reminiscence project called "Remembering Yesterday Caring Today (RYCT)", working on a project for eighteen weeks on education and themed reminiscence with people with dementia and their family carers. This resulted in being requested to be part of the European Research project to ensure reminiscence becomes recognised as a validated therapy in the future across the world once funds become available.

The RYCT project involved the use of artists, dramatists and musicians. Its main aims were simply to help find effective ways to preserve communication, sustain social relationships, support families and keep them in loving and caring relationships for as long as possible; rediscover pleasure through shared activities and have fun learning new skills together.

Its tremendous success in fulfilling its aims enabled us to run a "Magic Moments", living exhibition as a finale to the whole project. It gave the project members a chance to share some of their reminiscences with others in form of displays and tableaux depicting all the themes covered in the project e.g. Where we grew up, Schooldays, Courtship and marriage, Home-life, Wartime and Going to work. Its success has allowed it to be funded once again by Community Education (now Adult Learning and Leisure), to run for a second term and set up the reminiscence learning group for carers and those suffering from a dementia or memory difficulties.

National and European

Second Building Block

The second "networking" building block was my being asked to coordinate the South West Regional Reminiscence Network or REMNET as it has been officially named. It has a purple pansy as its logo, purple for reminiscence and a pansy for remembrance. REMNET will allow all those interested in the work of reminiscence to share best practice, meet socially and at fund-raising events, access assisted training workshops and conferences, communicate via e-mail, share resources and distribute a South West Newsletter to keep local people informed and up to date with local reminiscence information as well as national or European projects and news.

Although only in its infancy its membership continues to grow and it will soon be part of the Reminiscence Learning website.

Networking

Third Building Block

My third block and a larger block than the others, was the "training" block. It was a great privilege to be seconded for 2 years as the Reminiscence Therapy Trainer / Coordinator into Somerset Partnership NHS and Social Care Trust Training Department with my trustworthy friend and colleague Jacqui Cridge. Our main aim was to set up and run reminiscence training sessions within the Trust and voluntary and private sectors throughout the South West. Unfortunately a lack of funding prevented the secondment from going to term, but my passion and commitment to reminiscence unleashed in me the original drive and motivation I had experienced when this whole project started and therefore I had to continue with the reminiscence training in some form or another. After many months of planning, cogitating and deliberating, I finally decided to grasp the thistle and go it alone. So a new company was set up called Reminiscence Learning and another part of life's patchwork quilt was formed.

Reminiscence learning is now being run as a limited company, non-profit making and pending charitable status. It has a wide variety of courses available covering topics such as reminiscence, dementia care and activity and runs regular themed workshops on music and dance, traditional skills and crafts, libraries, archives and museums, and down on the farm, a rural workshop. (For more course details see end of this chapter).

It also has a reminiscence resource library for use by members. Our chartered librarian Birgit James explains in greater detail on page 79.

Training

Fourth Building Block

Building block number four represents "technology" the new computer system and software by comm@NET, which will enable us to store all community archive material, people's memories in the form of text, photographic, sound or video images. This is probably the most innovative and futuristic block focusing on the technology of the future.

Technology

Fifth Building Block

And finally the fifth building block is for "creativity". We have now created a second reminiscence centre at The British Legion Home, Dunkirk Memorial House, Bishops Lydeard, Taunton a much larger room and based on the 1940's and 1950's. Another very exciting challenge that has been gratefully put within my reach, and a project that I will endeavour to make as successful if not more so than the first Penny Farthing Reminiscence Centre in Wellington.

Creativity

But of course the future success is all thanks to the foundation building block that retains all these blocks resolutely together and allows the tower to soar ahead and reach further into the future becoming more resilient and powerful as it recruits others along the way on its road to success.

No 7 NOVEMBER 1999

Somerset Partnership *news*

The Newsletter for all staff working in the new NHS and Social Care Trust

REMINISCENCE CENTRE OPENS

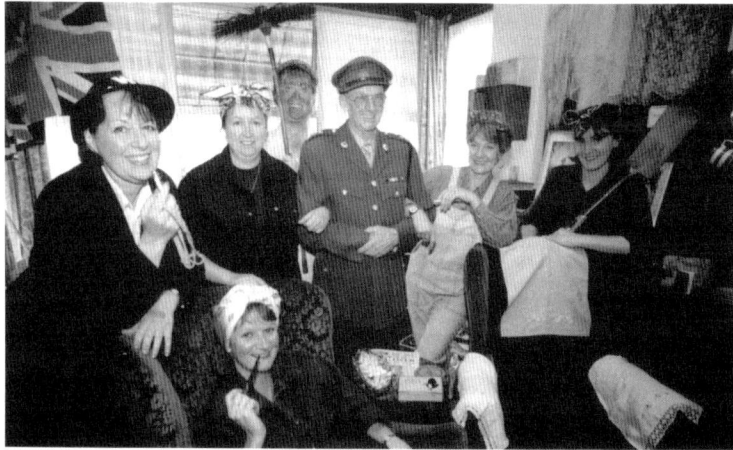

Remembrance Room: L to R back Carol Hart, Jaqui Cridge, Centa Stone, Trefor Wood, Patsy Trott, Sharon Hardie. Sitting is senior occupational therapist Fiona Mahoney.

THE NEWLY opened Penny Farthing Reminiscence Centre at Stratfield House in Wellington offers visitors the chance to step back in time to the 1930s and '40s.

This is a place where they can enjoy a cup of tea in a china cup of the type they might remember from childhood, while sitting around a period fire and playing parlour games.

'This room has been designed as a multi-sensory environment to offer visitors a hands-on experience,' said Senior Occupational Therapist Fiona Mahoney, who put the Centre together.

'We all reminisce in our own way, depending on our age or walk of life. This can be done formally in specialist groups, informally with a friend, relative or neighbour, or spontaneously as part of our everyday life experience. '

The Centre includes a fireplace, a war time corner, leisure and music section and a multi-sensory environment, together with lots of artefacts and memorabilia. There is also a place to sit and browse through old books, or just recall the past.

A weekly timetable has been drawn up which includes pre-booked sessions for schools, residential homes and hospital units.

**For further details contact Fiona Mahoney
phone 01823 661663**

NEWS ● VIEWS ● OPINIONS ● RESOURCES ● SUGGESTIONS ● ADVICE ● CONTACTS

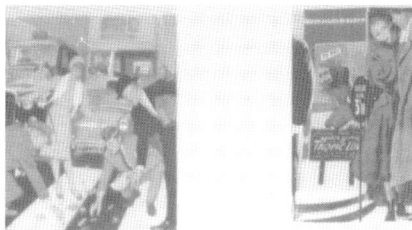

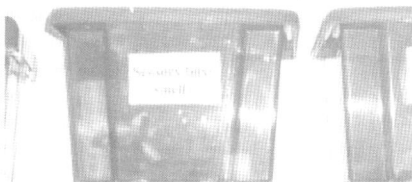

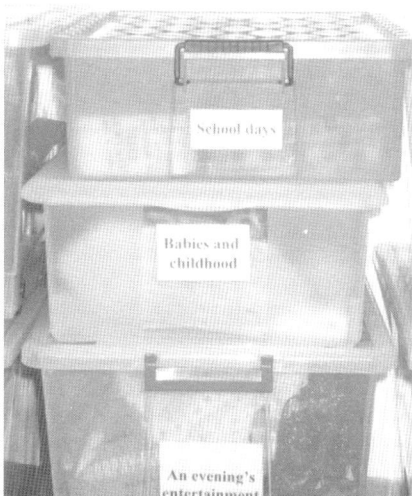

An important part of Reminiscence Learning is the library. There you can find books and other relevant resources for use in activities and for professional use by staff.

The library presently stocks over 200 books which cover a wide range of subjects. Some of the titles are covering areas such as local history, the Royal family, wartime history and memories, but also subjects like children's games, cookery books, crafts, poetry and transport are represented.

The library holds a large number of reminiscence theme boxes. These boxes are full of selected artefacts and memorabilia covering a particular subject. These themes include Childhood, Schooldays, Going to Work, Dressing up and looking good, Hats, caps and scarves, A day at the seaside and many more.

In each box are guidelines and ideas to enable you to get the best from your chosen box.

Many other types of resources are also in stock. There are items of clothing and outfits, fashion accessories, wigs and hats, games, jigsaw puzzles, newspaper packs, music on tape, CDs and records, audiotapes and videos. You can even use the candyfloss machine to ensure your seaside theme is even more realistic. Why not try it and see for yourself.

Sweets, pocket kites, Punch and Judy kits and lavender bags can also be purchased to use as part of your creative reminiscence activity.

We look forward to welcoming you as a member in the near future.

Birgit James
Chartered Librarian

Reminiscence

What is Reminiscence...Taster 2hr course

Volunteers and Carers Reminiscence package........................Introduction, theory and practical

Themed Reminiscence Workshops...Practical workshops (1day)

Music and Dance

Traditional Skills / Crafts

Down on the Farm / A rural workshop

Libraries, Museums and Archives

3* Reminiscence Package...Introduction to Reminiscence,
Theory and Practical
(2 day course)

4* Reminiscence Package...Intermediate Course
(3 day course)

5* Reminiscence Package...Comprehensive Course
(4 day course)

All courses have high practical element

Dementia Care Training

Focusing on dementia through communication and
activity...An insight into the effect of dementia
and associated problems, practical tips
and activities related to behaviour
(1 day course)

Yesterday, Today, Tomorrow...Comprehensive, interactive course looking
at dementia and its related behaviours
and how to manage them (2 day course)

Activity Courses

Therapeutic activity
" Does it just keep the person occupied?".........................Analysing activity, its use and ideas
(1 day course)

Other courses and conferences available (changing and updating on a regular basis)
New courses Intergenerational Reminiscence and How to set up a memory room

If you have a specific learning need please contact Fiona on 01823 431257

How to use
the Reminiscence Room

REMINISCENCE

Should create an
atmosphere of

Fun

Relaxation

&

Well-being

**Reminiscence should create
an atmosphere of:**

FUN
RELAXATION
WELL - BEING

This room has been designed as a multi-sensory environment, and the purpose is for it to be used as a hands-on experience.

We all experience reminiscence in our own way, whatever age or walk of life, and this can be done formally in specialist groups, informally with a friend, relative or neighbour or spontaneously as part of our everyday life experience.

We want you to use our specially designed room in the way you feel most comfortable. It should be positive and

83

provide a feeling of well being as well as occasionally allowing time to reflect on some of our more sad memories as we remember old family members and those not so happy times.

Please use the room to suit your own needs, for example

- *Spend some quiet time alone.*

- *Use one of the specific theme boxes at home, work or school, exploring topics such as:*

1. *Childhood and schooldays*

2. *Going to work*

3. *A day at the seaside*

4. *An evening's entertainment*

5. *Royalty*

- *Listen to some music, play a record of your choice.*

- *Use your senses, taste, touch, and smell the wide variety of items in the sensory drawers and cupboards.*

- *Open the boxes, drawers, cupboards, and explore for yourself the wide range of trinkets and memorabilia.*

- *Read the numerous newspapers, articles, books, diaries etc.*

- *Sit and play cards, dominoes, shove ha'penny or use the skipping rope and spinning top.*

- *Sit by the fire and chat with others about your own personal memories.*

- *Read through the old recipes.*

- *Try on the hats, gloves, scarves and bags.*

- *Fill in the reminiscence quiz.*

Whatever way you personally choose to spend your time reminiscing – most of all enjoy it.

Ways to help encourage conversation and interaction within the room

- Allow enough time to browse in silence if preferred.

- Do not show off your own knowledge.

- Focus on the senses taste, touch and smell. They will often trigger memories.

- Provide soft background music to prevent awkward silences.

- Encourage hands – on interaction with the artefacts in the room.

- Ask open / probing questions to encourage more detailed conversation. E.g. "Tell me how you would use this", instead of, "Did you ever use one of these?"

- Use non-verbal communication such as nodding head and eye contact to show they are worthy listening to.

- Listen with empathy and interest.

- Concentrate on the task in hand and do not become side tracked by something that is of interest to you alone.

- Be aware that sometimes memories trigger sad emotional responses. This does not necessarily mean that the experience has been bad or that they want to leave the room. Be guided by their own reactions and act on them accordingly and within your own professional guidelines.

A personal example of clinical evaluation and how the Penny Farthing Room has proved to be a positive outcome in client care for one individual

This lady Mrs A was in her 70's and regularly attended the day hospital. She suffered from a dementia and lived within a residential care setting. She had limited possessions within her room and had not taken part in regular daily living activities such as cooking, cleaning, ironing for some considerable time. Her behaviour during the day was very disturbed and agitated. Without intervention, she sat for no longer than 2-3 minutes before she would stand up from her chair and come over to ask a member of staff where she was, why she was there and when would she be going home. This pattern repeated itself every 2-3 minutes throughout the day. Each time she would react as though she had never spoken to you before and although she was satisfied with the response she had forgotten the answer by the time she had returned to her chair and consequently felt anxious, lost and bewildered within the next few minutes.

With full consent from the family we decided to see what difference it would make to her behaviour if we showed her a box of reminiscence artefacts and also take her into the Penny Farthing Reminiscence room.

In order for this to be a valued exercise, we decided to take Mrs A into the quiet room away from external interruptions. We set up a camcorder on a tripod and asked her if she was happy for us to video the session. In the room there was Mrs A, myself and Jacqui. Jacqui operated the video but took no part in the session.

For the first 5 minutes Mrs A and I sat together in silence to show what happened when she was not engaging in any activity, as though she were sitting in a lounge with another resident or client. As expected within 2-3 minutes Mrs A started to behave as she had done previously, becoming restless and finally asking the same questions as to why she was here. Each question was answered and then we sat together in silence again. Twice more she repeated the questions and again I responded appropriately. It felt very uncomfortable and awkward for me.

I then asked Mrs A if she would like to take part in some reminiscence activities and she instantly responded to the hurricane lamp that I took out of the Home life box. She started to initiate the conversation. Several more items were taken out of the box and each time she responded appropriately and with interest, talking about each object and answering questions. The smell of the fairy soap triggered a memory for her and although she could not remember the name of it without prompting she knew it was soap and it had a very familiar smell. The hurricane lamp especially triggered memories of her father going down the mines and she was able to describe his job and place of work in some detail, stating that going down the mines was a dangerous job. Throughout the short session of handling objects in the box Mrs A did not revert back to her disorientation or confusion but concentrated and engaged well in the activity, socially integrating and appearing to enjoy the experience.

I then asked Mrs A if she would like a cup of tea. She said she would and so I told her both Jacqui and I would leave the room. The video was left running and the Home life box left open beside her.

Initially she just sat quietly and then she started to look through the box. She took out the feather boa and found this fascinating. She stroked the feathers, blew them, put the boa around her neck and finally used it as a comforter on her shoulder and closed her eyes.

We of course woke her up when we returned to the room and she drunk her tea chatting and reminiscing asking only once where she was and why she was here.

After tea I asked Mrs A if she would like to come and look at the new Penny Farthing Reminiscence Room. On entering the room Mrs A instantly recognised items and was engaged in activity. She initiated conversation and showed interest by her actions. She talked about the heavy iron and the coal-scuttle, although she could not remember its name and required some prompting. She instantly recognised the

kitchen cabinet and pull down work top and described how it was used for rolling out pastry. Her first words on entering the room were, "Oh, is this a memory room?" and throughout her time in the room kept saying, "Oh, memories".

This short but most enlightening exercise shows how engaging someone in an activity, that uses long-term memory and is failure free, can change a person's behaviour and stimulate them.

In conclusion:

When not occupied or engaged in reminiscence Mrs A repeats herself, is confused and disorientated and unsettled.

When she is occupied and engaged in a reminiscence activity the conversation is very different. She initiates conversation, she appears settled, her body language shows her enjoyment and she is less confused.

Here are another few examples and stories from colleagues working within the day hospital setting and who have also experienced exciting and surprising results by using the Penny Farthing Reminiscence Centre in a variety of interesting and unusual ways.

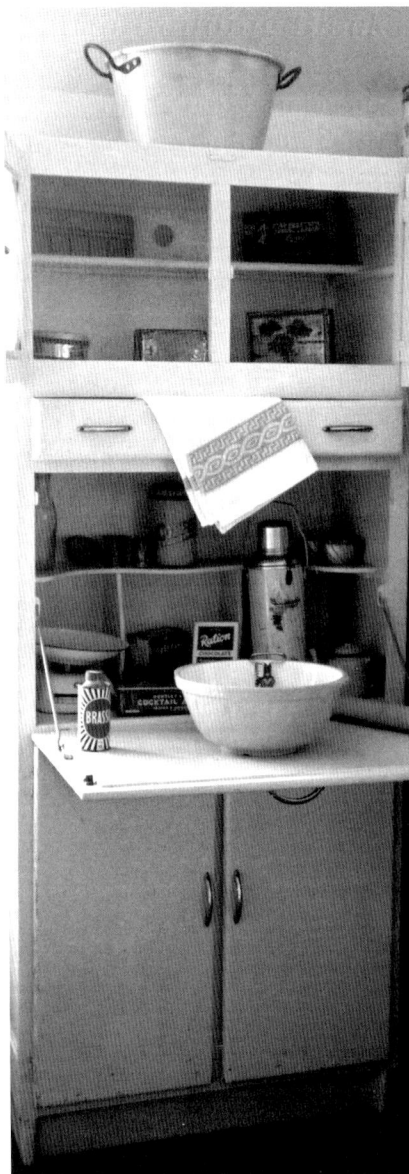

I have used the Penny Farthing Reminiscence room on many occasions in my role as a Staff Nurse in the Day Hospital and I would like to share with you two particular stories that sums up for me what a reminiscence room is all about.

Story 1

I provided counselling sessions for Bob, a deeply depressed gentleman who was struggling to come to terms with his diagnosis. I usually carried out these sessions in the quiet lounge of the hospital away from noise and distraction. Ten counselling sessions were provided and although by the seventh there was a definite improvement, I still struggled to find a 'feel good' factor that I could develop further and close the sessions on.

By accident the eighth session had to be provided in a different room. The only private and available room left was the Penny Farthing Reminiscence Centre, so I had no choice but to do the counselling there.

The instant I took Bob into this themed room I noticed a flicker of interest and excitement in his eyes, something that had been missing from his presentation since we first met. Bob spoke of remembering living in a house similar to the one he found himself standing in now, the smells that reminded him of his youth – mothballs and Brylcream. Bob commented on the kitchen cupboard, which he laughed at when it screeched as he pulled open the front pastry shelf. "They all make a sound like that," he told me. He set about showing me how to use the old Brownie camera and told me stories of travelling by steam train.

I allowed Bob a few moments to reflect on his memories the room had triggered before we continued with the counselling session, which proved to be the most productive, and forward moving I had experienced. Before leaving Bob asked if future sessions could be held in the same room and I saw no reason why they could not.

The next two sessions proved just as rewarding and Bob was eager to further explore the room so he could go back and tell his wife all about it. At long last he had something to talk about with his wife. Bob explained that the room had an atmosphere that was relaxing and comfortable for him and that made him feel quite at home.

It has stirred some happy memories and had provided a topic of extended conversation and interest when at home. This had reawakened his interest in life and as he chuckled at the old photographs and read extracts from the old newspapers he recalled his experiences of living through the era and told anecdotes of his childhood.

This room had now given Bob a purpose and that was to write a life story or start up an album of his life and share this with his grandchildren. In the interim he intended to bring his wife along to visit the room.

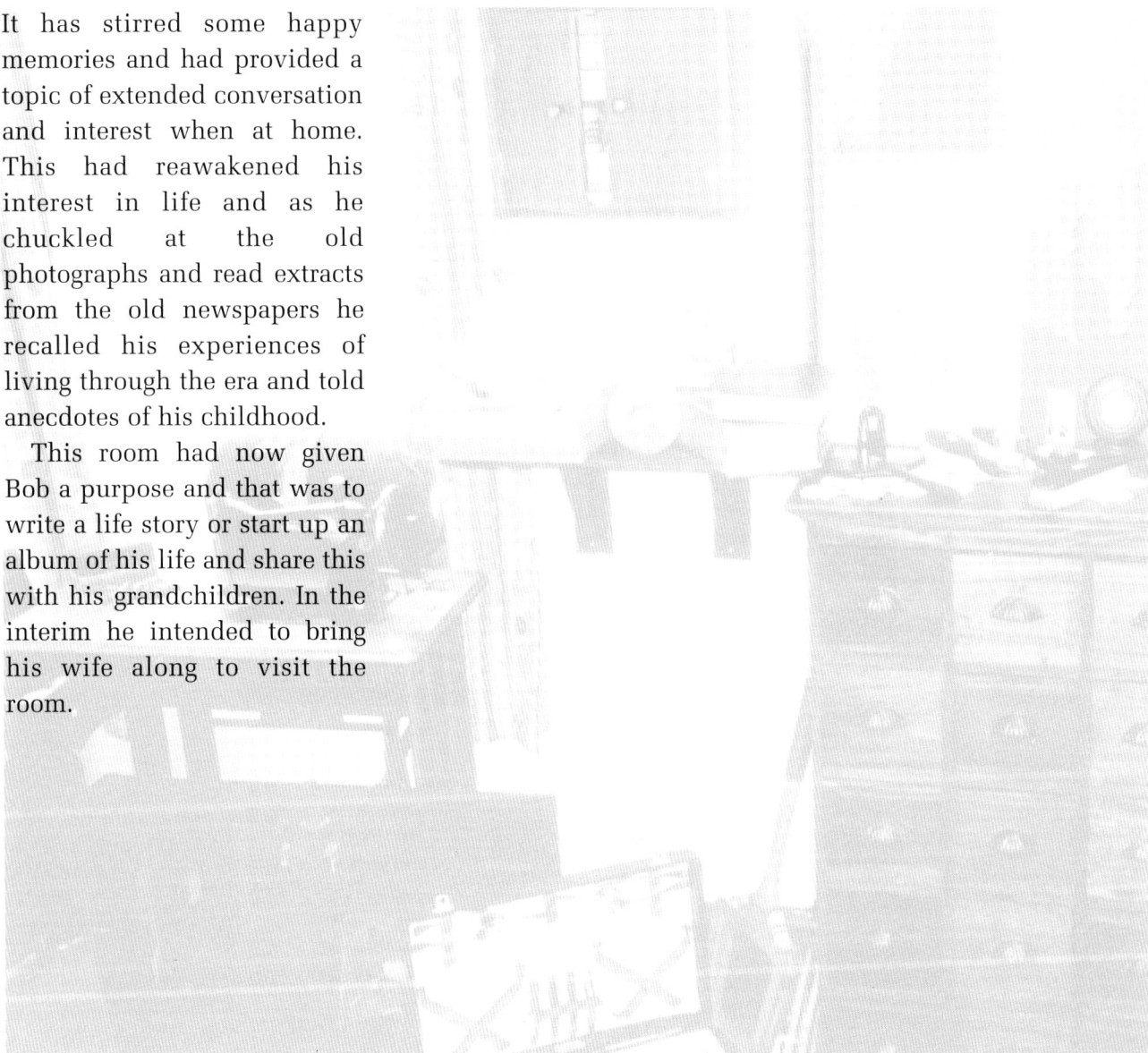

Story 2

I nursed two ladies who were diagnosed with dementia and often had difficulties relating conversation with the present day. One particular lady had lost all confidence in talking out as she feared she had nothing of interest to speak about, especially to people she didn't know well. I took these two ladies into the reminiscence room as part of their care programme and monitored the outcome.

Both ladies were amazed by the room and I instantly observed them talking of items in the room as being dated. This gave me the impression that they were orientated enough to recognise this room was not of the present era.

The ladies spoke fondly of stories of making pastry and rolling it out on the pastry shelf of the kitchen cupboard and they even exchanged recipes. They shared stories of war – one lady was in the land army and spoke of the war days as being happy times because of the community spirit. The tin helmets and newspapers of the declaration of the war in the war corner triggered this.

Both enjoyed an hour in the room of non stop chatting and reminiscence and even during dinner when they were no longer in the Penny Farthing Centre they spent the whole time reminiscing and swapping stories of their lives. Despite the afternoon sessions being largely interrupted by these two ladies who didn't stop talking about their experience in the room and their memories it had triggered, it was nice to see that they had something to talk about which boosted their confidence and morale. This left them going home later in the day feeling good.

Jacqui Cridge RMN

Story 3

I had a referral to see a lady who was suffering from anxiety and depression following a fall three years ago. She had become isolated, frightened to leave the house, and subsequently very low. I had basically tried everything possible to get to know her, and find out about her life and problems but could not get past the pain she was suffering in her back – this had become a reason to decline involvement in all activities on offer, and the reason she did no domestic or household activities. She refused to walk any distance even around the unit. I was at a complete loss, totally unable to form any rapport with her or even think of starting any treatment.

One day she agreed to walk around the unit with me, and didn't seem to be in much pain, or complaining of pain so to extend the distance I took her into the reminiscence room. Immediately on entering the room there was a difference in her. She became very relaxed, and started moving around the room picking things up. She told me what the items were and what she remembered being in her mother's house. She really opened up, especially when I showed I didn't know what most of the things were for!

It turned out that she had worked as a museum curator, and had been an active member of the archaeological society until her fall. We established a good rapport, and trust. She enjoyed teaching me things. This also went on to telling the group about her experiences around Exmoor. She was so relaxed with me at the end of the session; she walked back to Stratfield via outside, which was a major achievement. This then built up to walking into Wellington to visit the museum and visiting other museums.

I believe it played a large part in building her self-esteem, feeling of value, and self worth. She became a very interesting member of the day hospital group.

Melanie Leaver, Senior Occupational Therapist

92

Let's hope that by using reminiscence as a therapeutic activity either formally in groups or informally with an individual it will allow residents and clients to become less agitated and confused and provide the FUN, RELAXATION and WELL-BEING we aim to achieve.

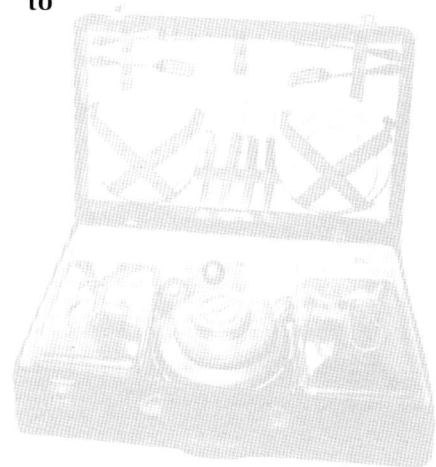

"Wicked!"

"The room, the smell, everything wonderful.
Just like going back in time. I'm coming back"

Fascinating Nostalgia

Wonderful!

"Really good smells, sounds. Could spend a long time looking at everything"

"Brings back happy memories"

Very interesting to see and touch

"Delightful display. A lovely experience"

A brilliant look back in time. Well done!

" I have been overwhelmed. The old memories flew back "

"I remember that from Grandma's house. Brings back memories"

Lovely Place

7.Where do you go from here?

You have now embarked on this reminiscence adventure and followed the memory-making trail. You are hopefully as excited and enthused as I was when I first stepped back in time at the Age Exchange Reminiscence Centre in London. You now have a little more insight into how to go about setting up your own room and some of the hazards and snares that may slow down your journey or trip you up along the way.

Believe me however easy it may all seem, when you first start to create your own vision, it is full of many pot-holes and boggy wasteland. But please do not despair-there is always light at the end of the tunnel and those who are determined enough in life will always fulfil their ambitions and dreams. I know because I did it. I feel very proud and, have a real sense of achievement so much so that I have now, as I touched on before, created a second room at Dunkirk Memorial House. So surely, it really can't be that bad. It's just like having a baby. You soon forget all the pain!

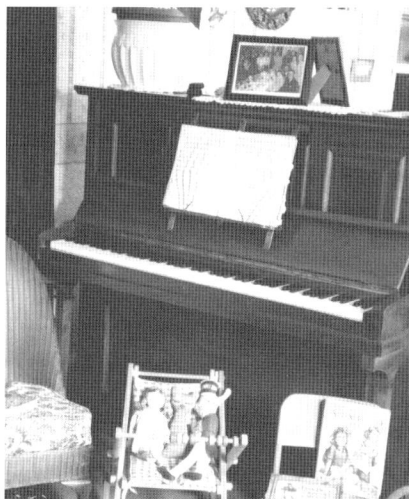

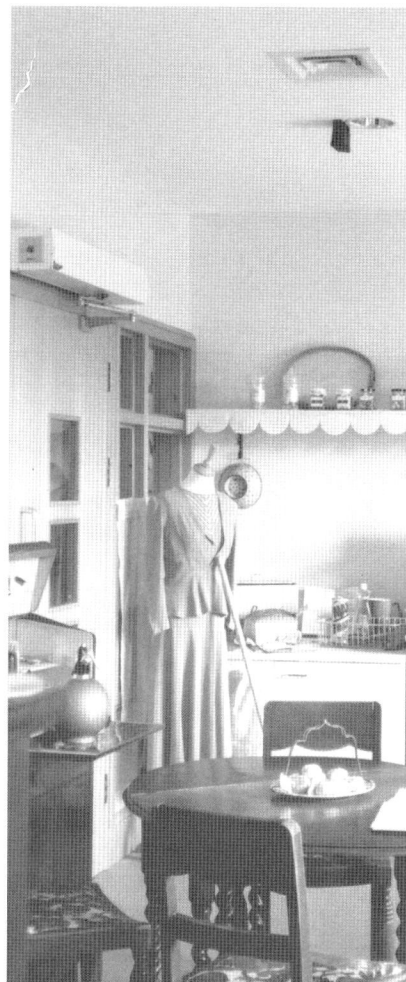

Perhaps you still feel you need to learn more about reminiscence. Perhaps you would like to visit the Penny Farthing Reminiscence Centre and see for yourself. Perhaps you'd like to hear it from the "horse's" mouth, so to speak. Well all these options are possible. As an occupational therapist now running my own training company, Reminiscence Learning, and still working with my friend and colleague Jacqui Cridge (RMN), we cover the South West, training people in the use of reminiscence with a variety of training packages. We also run tailor made packages and smaller half or one-day courses and regular conferences entitled "A positive approach to dementia" "An alternative approach for the use of reminiscence" and

"Setting up your own reminiscence room".

All courses have both a theoretical and practical element and are guaranteed to be enjoyable and fun. (see list of courses at end of chapter 5).

If you would like to be involved in the South-West Regional Reminiscence Network REMNET we would like to hear from you. A way we can share our skills, knowledge and resources to ensure best practice for reminiscence throughout the West Country.

And remember that once the adequate funding becomes available the University College London will be running a European Reminiscence Research Project of which we in Somerset have been invited to be part. This will enable reminiscence to at last become a validated and fully recognised therapy.

What do they say? "From little acorns, oak trees grow!"

However much you think you know about reminiscence, there is always more to learn. So never stop learning and remembering.

Top tips for setting up a reminiscence room

- Ensure you have a real interest and love of reminiscence. Research your subject, read lots of books and documents.

- Do not try to do it alone. You need a team of interested and committed people to share the numerous jobs.

- Speak to your family and close friends. They may well have a loft full of memorabilia or have memories and stories of their own memories that they wish to share.

- Your family will be involved. Allow them in, they are often needed during evenings and at weekends and you definitely need their sympathy, empathy and support.

- Research your chosen era well. It is so easy, as we have found from experience, to drift off 10 years ahead or 20 years before, without realising.

- Use the library for a list of reminiscence books and article research.

- Be clear about your aims for the room's use. Who you would like and trust to use it and approximately how many people can be in the room at one time.

- Choose your venue carefully. Ensuring it is large enough – because it is surprising how much you will collect over a period of time.

- Enlist artists, photographers, writers, interior designers etc.

- Start collecting photographs, reminiscence books, videos, newspapers, documents and old magazines early on. Purchase from book clubs, Past Times, junk shops, charity shops, car boot sales, antique shops and reclamation yards.

- Do a presentation to your local League of Friends, Alzheimer's Society, Social Services Departments, Arts development team.

- Have regular fund raising events early on to encourage the local community to be aware of your project. They will often provide many areas of help.

- Speak to your local newspaper. Encourage them to follow your story from the beginning even when it is just an idea. Invite them regularly to take photographs and write regular press releases and editorial. They will print this all free of charge. Fund raising events can also be put in the listings section at no cost to you.

- Don't be afraid to ask for money. Make sure you ask for enough. So prepare a budget in advance. It's surprising how many hidden costs there are.

- Keep a photographic record and diary for your archive. Buy albums and start to collate them from the beginning, It's easier to do this as you go along than to leave it until the end of the project. You probably won't do it then. Save letters, lists, drawings, sketches, material swatches and paint colours. Also keep a list of addresses and useful contacts, even if you don't use them all. They may be useful in the future.

- Always write and thank people for gifts donated for raffles etc and keep them informed of your progress. They are more likely to help next time.

- Don't be afraid to ask for donations. Polite cheek works. If you don't ask you don't get.

- Sometimes you will have to use replica furniture or not the genuine article but as long as it gives the right impression, don't worry.

- Be aware of health and safety and fire regulations. They often don't give you the answer you want but it's best to be aware from the beginning.

- Respect other people's memories and treasured possessions. If they decide to donate items to your centre, create a form for them to sign stating that the named item they are giving you is a gift and not on loan. This will prevent any embarrassment later on. (See Appendix 1)

- Display a disclaimer in the room. (See Appendix 2).

- All items in the room should be documented in a detailed itinery.

- If you have personally given items that you do not wish to become permanent fixtures, ensure this is well documented and counter signed.

- Choose a name that is catchy and doesn't sound like a second hand gift shop.

- Be ambitious with your choice of celebrity guest. There are often local celebrities who would be more than willing to take part.

- Continue to learn and improve your knowledge.

- Market the room and spend money on a professional brochure to promote your reminiscence centre.

- Finally enjoy yourself and have lots of fun creating a valuable space in which to treasure other people's memories. It's worth all the hard work. Believe me.

Name . . . .

Address . . . .

Telephone number . . . .

Description of item . . . .

. . . .

The Penny Farthing Reminiscence Centre is pleased to accept your donation on the understanding that the items donated are freely given for the organisation's use and they will not be needed. If this is acceptable please sign below:

Signature . . . .   Date . . . .

Would you like to receive a letter of acknowledgement?

Yes . . . .   No . . . .

(for official use only)

Acknowledgement sent by . . . .

Date . . . .

Item location . . . .

Please be aware that all items in this centre are old and therefore require careful handling as they may have sharp edges, rusty sides or may be very fragile.

Please therefore handle with care.

Thank you

National Association for Providers of activities for older people.
5, Tavistock Place,London
WC1H 9SN
0207 835757
www.napa.web.co.uk

Age Exchange Reminiscence Centre,
11, Blackheath Village,
London
SE3 9LA
0208 3189105
email:
administrator@ageexchange.org.uk
www.ageexchange.org.uk

Past Times
www.past-times.com

Wellington Weekly News
26 High Street, Wellington, Somerset
TA21 8RA

Bradfords Building Supplies,
Wellington New Road,
Taunton, Somerset
01823 254666

Otter Wrought Iron Products
12 Fourth Avenue
Bluebridge
Halstead, Essex
CO9 2SY
01787 475060

Spiller and Webber Ltd.
Builders Merchants
Victoria Street
Taunton, Somerset
01823 337333

Philip Knighton (The gramophone man)
17, South Street
Wellington, Somerset
01823 661618

Chris Levack
Comm@NET
PO Box 27
Leeds
LS13 1XS

REMNET
(Reminiscence network south west)
Patsy White / Fiona Fraser
01278 446165
or Fiona Mahoney
01823 431257

Penny Farthing Reminiscence Centre
Stratfield House
Bulford
Wellington, Somerset
TA21 8QQ
01823 661663

Somerset Virtual College NHS
Dunkirk Memorial House
Minehead Road
Bishops Lydeard
Taunton, Somerset
TA4 3BT
01823 431259

Reminiscence Learning (Training Courses and Resource Library)
Room 57
Dunkirk Memorial House
Minehead Road
Bishops Lydeard
Taunton, Somerset
TA4 3BT
01823 431257
email:
fiona@reminiscencelearning.co.uk

Take Art
Ralph Lister
email:
ralph.takeart@dial.pipex.com

Crump A (1997) "Room to Remember"
Nursing Practice Reminiscence
Elderly Care June/July **Vol 9 NO3**

Gibson F (1994) *"Reminiscence and Recall"*
England: Age Concern

Kitwood T (1997) *"Dementia Reconsidered"*
Buckingham: Open University Press

Osborn C (1993) *"The Reminiscence Handbook"*
London: Age Exchange

Schweitzer P (1998) *"Reminiscence in Dementia Care"*
London: Age Exchange

Suggested Reading List

Department of Health (2001)
"National Service framework for older people"

Kitwood T and Bredin K (1992) *"Person to person"*
Bradford Dementia Group: Bradford University

Sim R (1997) *"Reminiscence - Social and creative activities"*
Derbyshire: Winslow Press

Journal of Dementia Care
London: Hawker Publications

Best of British (past and present)
Lincolnshire: Ian Beacham Publishing
www.bestofbritish.co.uk

List of Thanks

I would like to thank all my colleagues, family and friends for all their support and help throughout this whole ambitious project.

Especially those involved in the steering group namely Tracey Bright, Mandy Knight, Helen Mcevansoneya and Lin Symons for all her long hours typing, Jacqui Cridge for her dedication and long hours spent with me setting up, cleaning and organising the room and who read my original draft. Also to Steve Bellringer for the number of maintenance hours he spent in the room, and to Lyn Ferguson for her knowledge of colours and interior design. Thank you also to the Wellington Cottage Hospital League of Friends for their monetary support and general optimism in the project, Somerset Partnership NHS Social Care Trust for allowing me to use my skills as an occupational therapist to develop and formulate these ideas.

Age Exchange, especially Pam Schweitzer whose continual enthusiasm and encouragement helped me through the choppy waters.

The local suppliers, Spiller and Webber and Bradford Building Supplies, who supplied materials and the local community including the Wellington Weekly newspaper who followed the story from its initial conception.

Thank you to my script readers namely Karen Symon who kindly assisted me with my english grammar. My sister Trina who has always been a source of inspiration and support and constructively criticised my script with tender but poignant sisterly love and my true friend Bee James who has read and re-read my script and has spent many enjoyable hours with me over many a cup of coffee.

Not forgetting David Waddilove and the Somerset Virtual College NHS who chose to have faith in publishing this book.

However it is my husband Ken who has probably been the most patient and long suffering of them all, never doubting my abilities, always sharing in my ideas and being there as my resource for dates. Always giving of his free time at weekends, evenings and holidays and when I had another mad idea and had to, in my true Taurean nature, act upon it immediately.

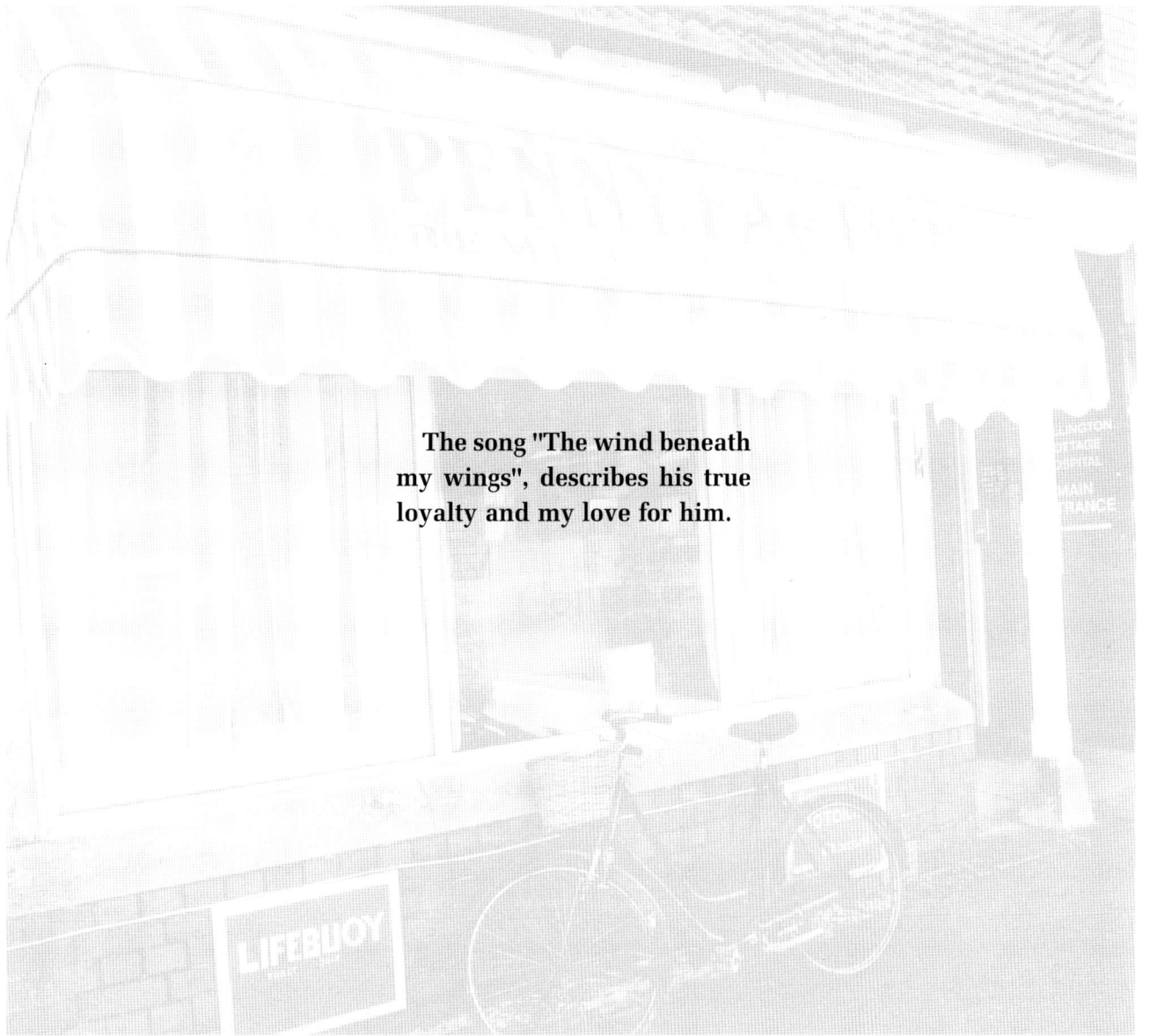

The song "The wind beneath my wings", describes his true loyalty and my love for him.